The Power That Heals

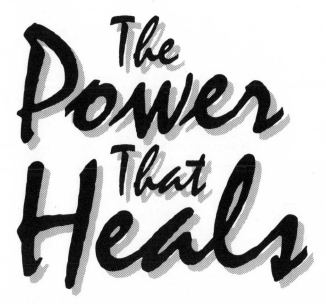

The Power That Heals

Love, Healing & The Trinity

DAVID JAMES RANDOLPH

Abingdon Press
Nashville

THE POWER THAT HEALS:
LOVE, HEALING, AND THE TRINITY

Copyright © 1994 by Abingdon Press

This book is printed on recycled, acid-free paper.

Library of Congress Cataloging-in-Publication Data

Randolph, David James, 1934-
    The power that heals: love, healing, and the trinity/by David
James Randolph.
        p.   cm.
    Includes bibliographical references.
    ISBN 0-687-33207-9 (alk. paper)
    1. Health—Religious aspects—Christianity. 2. Medicine—
Religious aspects—Christianity. 3. Trinity. I. Title.
BT732.R26   1994
261.5′61—dc20   93-31888
                                                                                      CIP

Scripture quotations, unless otherwise noted, are from the New Revised Standard Version Bible, Copyright © 1989 by the Division of Christian Education of the National Council of the Churches of Christ in the USA. Used by Permission.

Those noted KJV are from the King James, or Authorized, Version.

94 95 96 97 98 99 00 01 02 03 — 10 9 8 7 6 5 4 3 2 1

MANUFACTURED IN THE UNITED STATES OF AMERICA

To Joey and Cindy Adams,
Lovers and Healers

CONTENTS

ACKNOWLEDGMENTS

It may seem a simple thing, having written a book, to acknowledge the help of others and to thank them. Actually this has been a moving and, at times, overwhelming experience because it has made me aware of the people who have helped and still help me along my way. To them all I am deeply grateful, and especially to those who have contributed to this project.

My hearty thanks to:

Joey and Cindy Adams. Joey has generously shared his great faith, insight, healing humor, and encouragement with me. Cindy, the Oracle of Fifth Avenue, looked over an early chapter and made helpful suggestions from her rich storehouse of faith and practice.

Dr. David H. C. Read, former pastor at Madison Avenue Presbyterian Church in New York City, who took time to read a draft of this work and make suggestions. David was my neighbor in the city for years, and I remember not only his superb preaching but also running into him from time to time on hospital calls, a vital part of ministry.

Dr. Olin Ivey, who brought his bright learning to the reading of a draft. His discussion was illuminating.

Grace Geiger, who worked on an earlier version of this manuscript.

Lisa Hoffman, who processed the manuscript for publication and went above and beyond the call of duty in responding to what she was typing and encouraging me along the way.

Alexander Lowen, M.D., my analyst, teacher, and colleague, who has helped me with many of these issues.

Norman Cousins opened up a vast new territory. I was fortunate enough to receive his personal invitation to enter it when he came to Christ Church, Manhattan, and later corresponded with me.

Stephan Rechtschaffen, M.D., for his teaching and practice, and his colleagues at Omega Institute, which is also an Alpha for me, a place of beginnings.

Kurt Vonnegut, who continues to teach me about writing and living.

Daniel J. Travanti, for telling me what it was like to recover before it became fashionable to do so.

Sam Keen, who encouraged me on the Outlaw path.

Joseph Campbell, whose heroic study of the power of myth quickened my interest in the power of faith.

Rabbi Arthur Schneier, President of the Appeal of Conscience Foundation, which demonstrates the power of faith in international affairs.

John Cardinal O'Connor invited me to be a part of his committee on substance abuse. We didn't agree on everything, but we agreed that at the heart of the problem of addiction is a spiritual vacuum that only faith can fill.

Bishop Forrest C. Stith of the New York area of The United Methodist Church, who leads with a healing touch.

The Reverend William H. Perkins, Jr., the Reverend Clayton Z. Miller, the Reverend Noel Koestline, and the Reverend Pat Townsend, who are all capable executives and caring persons.

Bishop Dale and Gwen White, who encourage me by word and deed.

Ira Progoff, for sharing with me and others his Intensive Journal process.

My support group, which does support.

Edward Lawrence Hoffman. Ed's ministry to me and my family, especially to my father, in a time of crisis introduced me to the healing power of faith. His friendship across the years still helps.

To those medical doctors and health practitioners who have helped me toward healing.

To Diane Zemba, D.C., for helping me to a more vital understanding of affirmation and wellness.

The members and friends of The United Methodist Church in Babylon. They minister to me in my ministry to them and teach me much.

Carol O'Hanlon, my associate, is a caring person as well as a colleague.

The Affirmation Group of Babylon. These dear ones are the living laboratory for much of this material.

The members and friends of Christ Church United Methodist, Manhattan, where much of this approach was developed.

Linda Trichter-Metcalf and Tobin Simon, of whom I think and thank.

Many of my teachers have been with me in spirit as I have worked, encouraging me after all these years: Carl Michalson, Paul Tillich, Paul Schilling, Allan Knight Chalmers, Nels F. S. Ferre.

Stanley Romaine Hopper was my mentor for more than thirty years, opening his mind, his heart, and with Helen, his home. I am grateful to him for discussion of themes fundamental to this book that took place not only in classrooms but also at other great theological institutions, such as Yankee Stadium on that unforgettable Mickey Mantle Day.

To my family I am especially grateful. My father, my mother, and my brother Harry have crossed over the bridge between life and death, but still they speak to me in words that cannot be uttered.

Joy, my sister, and Jack, my brother, who in different ways teach me more than they can know.

Dave, my son, and Tracey, my daughter, have lived through much of this with me, and the experience of love that goes beyond all definitions has grown with them.

I say with D. H. Lawrence, "Look! We have come through!"

I am deeply grateful to all those who have shared their stories with me and made my story more meaningful. The persons and events I describe here are real, but some names have been changed for the sake of confidentiality.

I have sought to use inclusive language throughout this book. As to the Trinity itself, which refers historically to God as Father, Son, and Holy Spirit, it is worthy of note that some of the best thinking on the Trinity is coming from feminist theologians. While the doctrine of the Trinity was shaped in a patriarchal era, it does not have to be interpreted in a patriarchal way. I hope my approach here will do justice both to the historical formulation and to the emerging situation.

PREFACE

The health care crisis is the major challenge today because it raises the fundamental questions What is health? and Who cares?

The crisis is economic, but it is also spiritual. Unless the latter is recognized, the costs will spiral even higher, for it is estimated that the majority of people who seek medical help in America today are suffering from stress-related disorders. The cost of treating behavior-related diseases such as heart ailments, pulmonary diseases, and eating disorders by traditional means is in the billions of dollars, and the cost of dealing with HIV/AIDS is staggering as well. The human cost is beyond calculation. Moreover, the crisis within the health care professions is so great that many people no longer have confidence in them, and many professionals feel under attack and demoralized.

As desperate as the crisis is, there are resources for dealing with it. One is the emerging phenomenon that may be called spirit-body medicine, which builds upon mind-body medicine but proceeds from a spiritual base. The very titles of recent books by medical doctors and researchers suggest the major shift that is taking place: *The Spirituality of the Body* by

Alexander Lowen, M.D., *Quantum Healing* by Deepak Chopra, M.D., *Love, Medicine and Miracles* by Bernie Siegel, M.D., *The Faith Factor* by Herbert Benson, M.D., *Healing with Love* by Leonard Laskow, M.D., *Fire in the Soul* by Joan Borysenko, Ph.D., and the list can be extended. There are significant differences as well as agreements among these authors, but they share a more spiritual approach to the body that has far-reaching implications for theory and practice.

This spiritual approach to the body is not another "health fad" but a new expression of an old concern. "Are you practicing medicine or religion?" Bill Moyers asked Dr. Jon Kabat-Zinn during an interview for Moyers's popular television series "Healing and the Mind." "It depends on what you mean by medicine and what you mean by religion," replied Dr. Kabat-Zinn, explaining how the line between them is blurred. Although medicine and religion are separated in their narrow definition, he continued, "health comes from a root associated with 'whole' and 'holy' as well as 'heal,' so there's already a tie-in between religion and medicine."[1]

Excellent as this television series is, and the book based on it, the relationship between medicine and religion is expanding so rapidly that further studies are needed.

The purpose of this book is to contribute to this dialogue in a way that is informative and useful. I call for a new alliance between religion and medicine, focusing here on Christian faith but drawing attention to the resources of all the world religions. This way offers no panaceas. In fact, this way is hard, and its disciplines are demanding. Yet, those who follow it may find hope and healing.

It is my hope that our health care crisis will become a time of opportunity, and the fundamental questions stated above will be answered by those who declare: "Health is the movement from illness to wholeness, and we care!"

CHAPTER
ONE

THE JOURNEY TO WHOLENESS

"Do you want to be healed?" a great physician asked a partially paralyzed man. In the interview that followed, the man disclosed his desire, and the physician revealed the power that enabled the man to live his life in a new way. The man testified to what had happened, and an uproar occurred.

This case was reported years ago in the Gospel of John (5:1-18) and is reenacted today when physicians and their colleagues observe the power of healing and vigorously discuss "love, medicine, and miracles." The scientific recognition of faith and love as major factors in health is as momentous as the discovery of the atomic bomb and may yet unleash an implosion of life and healing greater than the explosion of death and disease. This book explores the power of love and the process of healing to the end that individuals and groups may move by faith and love toward wholeness.

Do you want to be healed? This is a personal question that cannot be answered in an abstract way. Therefore, you are invited to make your own journey toward wholeness throughout this discussion. At times, we will explore concerns that may seem to lack direct relevance to our theme. In the end, I hope their significance will become clear, but I will include suggestions to show the relevance of the material and to provide resources for integrating the insights into your experience.

Love heals. Have faith, and you may become whole. I confess that I was skeptical when introduced to these claims. Indeed, taken out of context, they are absurd. However, as I have studied them in the context of ancient religion and modern medicine, I am convinced that these claims are true, although they have a variety of meanings.

Modern medicine and religious tradition are converging around these themes. This book is about this revolutionary development. With the awareness that you may have a personal interest in how this convergence may affect you, I have sought to relate my subject to one who wants to move toward well-being. Those who have taken up the journey witness to its value—from the ancient paralytic to the contemporary pitcher, Orel Hershiser.

Winning the World Series and appearing on "The Tonight Show" are fantasies for most people. Disappointment and pain are reality. Orel Hershiser knows all of these experiences. He also knows that the God who creates, redeems, and sustains us can be a healing constant in the high moments of our triumphs and the deep moments of our despair.

Hershiser was the star of the 1988 World Series when he pitched the Los Angeles Dodgers to victory. There was a mystery when at one critical moment the star left the mound and prayerfully sang a song. But he came back, and he came through to win the game. Hershiser was an international celebrity, but he retained his modesty even when he appeared on "The Tonight Show." Johnny Carson asked Hershiser what song he had sung in the critical moment, but Hershiser was reluctant to answer. Carson persisted, and Hershiser finally sang in a light but firm tenor what he had sung in that game:

> Praise God from whom all blessings flow,
> Praise Him all creatures here below.

16

Praise Him above ye heavenly host,
Praise Father, Son and Holy Ghost.

This may have been the first time the doxology was sung on late night network television, but it was no oddity for Hershiser, whose faith in the Trinity is a major factor in his life. Not long after his great success, Hershiser suffered a tear in the labrum capsule of his pitching arm, which threatened to cripple him and end his career. But with surgery, therapy, and faith, he went through a long, hard rehabilitation. When he returned to the mound at Dodger Stadium in May of 1991, a huge crowd rose in a standing ovation.

Hershiser said, "I just thank God that this has all worked out and that I'm going to have another chance. . . . There's a lot of credit due in a lot of different places." He went on to thank his surgeon, the team physician, and the team therapist, who encouraged him day in and day out. He concluded, "To work as long and as hard as we have for thirteen months and go through the ups and downs, the one constant has been that God has been looking over us and has reassured us the whole time that something positive was going to come out of this."[1]

What happened to Orel Hershiser is not an isolated event but evidence of a power that is available to everyone: the power of love. In this book I set forth a connection between love, faith, and healing and offer a way to vitalize this connection and put it to work for us. Central to the book is a discussion of how faith as a body of belief contributes to the belief of a body. Specifically, we will explore how faith in the Trinity—God in three persons creating, redeeming, and sustaining—relates to health and wholeness. In reality, the very nature of the Trinity as wholeness means that the relation of the divine to humanity is healing—luring us to health and wholeness. Love is the key because God is love, loving us through creation, redemption, and sustenance and enabling us to love God, ourselves, and our neighbor into the wholeness that is health and salvation.

PREPARING FOR THE JOURNEY

Before we embark on this journey together, it may be helpful for me to share my definitions of key terms used throughout the book.

Love. It is important to define what we mean by love because the word is open to so many interpretations and all too often may pass for its complete opposite, as with the abusive parent who boasted that he "loved" his child so much that he beat him every night.

At the same time, love exceeds all our definitions. The effort to define *love* is most frustrating because what we are really looking for is not the definition of *love* but the experience of it. My hope is not to perfect a definition but to point the way to the reality of loving. Of how love heals we will say more as we proceed, but we may say that love is both the end and the means of healing.

Love is both a noun and a verb. Both aspects must be acknowledged and held together. As a noun, *love* refers to the passion *(eros)* and compassion *(agape)* that are directed toward other persons. As a verb, *love* refers to the acts by which passion and compassion are expressed. It is important to hold both the noun and the verb usages together, for if *love* is considered only as a noun, it lacks concreteness; if considered only as a verb, it lacks content. My understanding of love links passion and compassion with content and concreteness. The John who wrote "God is love" also wrote "In this is love, not that we loved God but that he loved us" (1 John 4:10). The love of God revealed in Jesus Christ is the ultimate definition.

Faith is the power to go on with our lives because of what we think, feel, imagine, and do in spite of everything that would turn us back. Christian faith is the power to go on with our lives because of what we think, feel, imagine, and do

18

about the God revealed in Jesus Christ as Creator, Redeemer, and Sustainer. For me, faith is venture; it is multidimensional and dynamic. It is also, paradoxically, small and common, available to us all with a power that may appear as modest rather than grand. It is not unusual in matters of ill health for faith to seem so insignificant as to be overlooked until more impressive medical routines are exhausted. Then the power that has always been there may be revealed as the decisive factor. Hebrews 11:1-13 is the classical expression of faith as "the assurance of things hoped for, the conviction of things not seen" and the pilgrimage to which we are called.

Health has usually been defined as the absence of disease. This view is seriously challenged today for its narrowness and negativity. The World Health Organization made a major redefinition of *health* in 1940 when it said that health is "a state of complete physical, mental and social well-being." To put it simply, we may say that health is not the absence of illness but the presence of wellness. Wellness is being in functional harmony with one's body, mind, spirit, and social setting. Wellness involves a regimen that includes regular check ups, consistent medical care, proper nutrition and exercise, as well as spiritual practices such as meditation. Wholeness also refers to the healthy harmony in which one's full resources are gathered with integrity. The words *health, wholeness,* and *wellness* are used interchangeably throughout this book.

Healing and Curing. These two words must be distinguished from each other. *Curing* refers to the correction of a medical or psychological dysfunction. A cure is possible in some cases, but not all. *Healing* can occur whether or not there is a cure of a particular ailment, because healing is the process by which we move toward wellness. Wholeness may involve not the total elimination of a problem but the ability to go on with one's life in spite of it.

In stressing the healing dimension of faith, I do not mean to suggest that faith is reducible to healing. Healing is only

19

an element of faith, albeit a central one. It is set within the context of the overall mission of the church to which Jesus called us in his Great Commission:

> Go therefore and make disciples of all nations, baptizing them in the name of the Father and of the Son and of the Holy Spirit. ... And remember, I am with you always, to the end of the age. (Matt. 28:19, 21)

Faith, Love, and Healing. How these three key terms are related to one another by the Trinity is the subject of this book. It is my conviction that faith gives us access to love, which brings healing.

The scientific recognition of love as an active force in wellness is a major breakthrough in medical research. A growing body of research identifies love as a variable in healing even though the precise definition of terms and functions is under study.

Healers on Healing is a collection of essays in which some of the world's leading healers explore their professional and personal experiences to uncover the principles on which healing rests. The editors find:

> Love is seen as one common denominator that underlies and connects all successful healing. Without it, there can be no true healing. For healing means not only a body without disease or injury, but a sense of forgiveness, belonging and caring as well.[2]

In this book we will show through personal anecdotes and scientific reports the validity of this conclusion as we seek to clarify terms, relate them to theology, and show their practical usefulness.

Spirituality and Religion. Much is made of the distinction between spirituality and religion. This distinction is valid because spirituality, by definition, relates to the spirit, which is numinous and otherworldly and universal. Religion, on the other hand, is that which seeks connection between the otherworldly and this world in a way that holds them together (the root is the Latin *religare*, "to bind together").

What is not much observed is that both spirituality and religion have positive and negative connotations. In the current literature under discussion, spirituality is treated largely as good in and of itself, while religion tends to be associated with institutions and dogma—and restrictive ones at that. In fact, spirituality, when not well grounded, can easily become spiritism, which means anything its practitioner wants it to mean. And while religion may be sick, it may also be healthy, as William James observed in his classic and still relevant *Varieties of Religious Experience*.

It was healthy religion to which Carl Jung referred when he observed that after treating people from all over the world for thirty years he had not seen one in the second half of life (over thirty-five) "whose problem in the last resort was not that of finding a religious outlook on life."[3] This, of course, had to do not with a particular creed or church but with that essential connectedness that religions have given to those who follow them.

More study is needed in this area. While it is necessary to distinguish between spirituality and religion, it is also necessary to recognize healthy and unhealthy varieties of each and to develop that which is healthy in both. John Bradshaw deals directly and creatively with this issue in *Creating Love* (see esp. his chap. 9 on the love of God).

MY STORY

Do you want to be healed? The will to be healed does not guarantee the result. But without the will, healing cannot occur. "Yes," you may answer immediately, "of course." Everyone hurts somewhere and would like to find relief. But do you *really* want to be healed? Are you willing to do what is required to be well, or have you, like the paralytic, gained a payoff from your paralysis?

The step from paralysis to power is enticing, but it is not easy. Our wounds are to the soul as well as to the body, as D. H. Lawrence wrote:

I am not a mechanism, an assembly of various sections.
And it is not because the mechanism is working wrongly,
    that I am ill.
I am ill because of wounds to the soul, to the deep emotional
    self
and the wounds to the soul take a long, long time, only
    time can help
and patience, and a certain difficult repentance
long, difficult repentance, realization of life's mistake, and
    the freeing oneself
from the endless repetition of the mistake
    which mankind at large has chosen to sanctify.[4]

I know this from my own experience. While it is not possible here to give the details of my medical history, it may be helpful to share a pattern I discovered that may be called "an anatomy of a recovery."

When I was in my second year of college, I came down with a serious illness and was forced to leave school. I was diagnosed with a chronic infection, and when I sought the opinion of a specialist from a famous hospital, he found a blockage in my system that could not be treated surgically and was sure to cause further complications.

It is now many years since that winter of my illness. I still ache with the memory of it. Although wounded like Jacob after wrestling with the stranger in the night who turned out to be an angel, I was able to limp into the future.

I feel that just to be alive is a gift of grace. This feeling is very deep, and even now I cannot handle it or articulate it very well. And yet my life is an attempt to do just that: to affirm that however desperate our situation may appear, we may live by faith, be saved by grace, and be empowered by God's love.

As I look back on that winter, I remember no one dramatic event that changed everything. There was none. I do remember a number of events, small in themselves, that helped to get me on the road again. One was finally giving in to despair, giving up, refusing to struggle anymore, accepting. I remember one night when a few stars of hope that had shone in my life—the calling I dreamed of, the young woman I loved, the very sense of the future—became extinguished. One by one they went out until only the darkness remained.

At that point, even the star of faith went out. The God who had been the God of my past, if indeed he had been God, was not the God of my present and could not be the God of my future, since I thought I had none. That God died, or more accurately, vanished. He just did not show up when I needed him most. My feeling was something like "God, if there is a God, which I seriously doubt, your will be done." That's it. I sank into the darkness.

I remember no immediate response to that. But as I look back on it, I believe that the darkness was a necessary prelude to the light that began to dawn, however dimly. I died that night—to my hopes and dreams and ambition. But I was not yet ready for a resurrection.

Another moment came later when I was reading the Psalms. I came across the verse "I will not die but live." I felt these words were addressed to me. Yes, I will live now. No, I will not die now. It was like a spontaneous, angry affirmation. But it stood alone as an act of will without a program to express it.

Through all this my family was supportive. My father, my sister, and my brothers were there for me in so many words and ways. That made it more difficult for me in some ways—but I could not let them down. My mother especially showed me love—love as close to the unconditional love of God as I had ever experienced. If I got well, she would love me. If I didn't get well, she would love me. But she believed I would get well. She told me a story about a wild duck that had become crippled. It had to stay out of the sky for a while, and that was a sad time. But the duck got well again and, one day, flew off. That would happen to me, she said. She believed that. I did not. I saw only my crippled wing and not the sky.

Then the pastor of our local church asked if I would like to teach a Sunday school class for children. It seemed like such a small and insignificant thing to do, far short of my lofty ambitions. I was not sure I could do it, or that I wanted to do it, but I felt I could try. I would take one small step back into the world. I took that step. I said yes. Right after a session from that class, a very lonely, frightened little girl came to talk to me. She was troubled. My heart went out to her. I said something she found helpful. She was grateful. I was alive.

In the spring of that year the pastor asked me to take on more responsibilities for the summer. I didn't know whether I could do it, but I felt somehow that I could try. I said yes. That summer I preached in my home church while the pastor was on vacation. One Sunday there happened to be in the congregation the pastor of one of the largest and most influential churches in the area. He was favorably impressed by my sermon. He invited me to visit him, and later he invited me to join his staff as a student minister. That was an opportunity beyond what I could have hoped for. My wing was still crippled, but suddenly I could see the sky. Ever since then the word *grace* has had a special meaning for me, for in that fellowship I found the grace to go on with my life.

I entered a nearby university. I got another diagnosis from a specialist who was more hopeful. His hopefulness increased mine. My health problems did not leave me, but they became chronic rather than acute. But there comes a time when one decides whether to remain an invalid or, like the paralytic by the pool, take up one's life and walk. When I found that I would never be cured, I found the grace to go on because I was not.

24

I did not know it at the time, but this crisis was my "initiation" into my life work. I still feel hurt, but many years later I can accept my wound as a gift.

It has been a continuing journey with descents into the depths and ascents into the heights. Lately, I feel more like I am moving with the flow of the air, although my wing still hurts at times. My life has not been a constant, upward flight since that time but a continuing journey instead.

THE JOURNEY TO WHOLENESS

The journey to wholeness involves four major movements, which I will simply identify here and develop as we proceed: awareness, acceptance, action, and affirmation.

Awareness. The journey to wellness begins with awareness. What are you aware of at this moment? In your body? In your mind? Where do you hurt? Where do you feel good? Consciously scan your body for points of pain or pleasure. What is the feeling? Where is it? In the stomach? In the head? Is it emotional? Do you feel guilty, ashamed, glad? Where is this feeling manifesting itself in your body?

Acceptance. Accept what you find whether you like it or not. Do not deny it. Surprisingly, much difficulty arises at this point. A person is aware, often vaguely, of pain or discomfort. But he or she dismisses it. Recently I visited a man in the hospital who had had a heart attack. In fact, he had been experiencing pains for some time but had dismissed them as "gas." His visit to the hospital, therefore, was for an attack that tore away part of his heart rather than for tests that might have led to treatment. Acceptance means recognizing that the pain is an indicator of some disorder that needs attention, not suffering in silence.

Action. Act to get at the root of the disorder and deal with it. Here a vast range of options is open to you. A medical examination and a second opinion are generally advisable. Alternative medicine may be sought. If a headache is clearly stress related, meditation may be called for. If it is related to a neurological disorder, another route is called for. But action is necessary.

Affirmation. Affirmation means saying yes to yourself and to life no matter what your condition is. It means choosing life rather than death. It means believing deeply that you will not die but live. Affirmations, statements in which we express these convictions, are likely to prove helpful. But affirmation itself underlies all these expressions and, in a sense, "begins" as well as "ends" the movements because affirmation deepens one's awareness.

The journey to wellness tends to ascend and descend, spiraling backward and forward on itself at different levels. Do not expect it to be a continuous, unbroken forward movement. There will be regressions as well as progressions. Also, the map of the territory reveals a fundamental pattern that will recur.

Wholeness is where we are going, and becoming whole is the way we go. Wholeness—more wellness, better health, affirmative living—is the vision toward which we journey. Wellness is not necessarily a cure in the sense of the removal of all traces of illness but the ability to move on with one's life whether or not a cure occurs. There may be the removal of physical difficulties, but wellness is demonstrated not by the absence of symptoms but by the presence of the ability to proceed toward the goals the person has chosen.

Wholeness (wellness) is not an escape from pain and suffering. Wellness implies not the elimination of pain and suffering but their embrace into a larger context that incorporates them into the functions of a whole person.

The poet e. e. cummings said that the goal of life is not to succeed but to proceed. This applies to our health as well. The goal of health is not to succeed in attaining an absolutely perfect state but to proceed toward a harmonious relationship with oneself, with other people, and with God. Let us proceed.

CHAPTER
T W O

AFFIRMATIVE LIVING

Do you believe in God? This question does not come up often in our ordinary lives where we are more likely to ask what we ought to be doing at the time. But in those moments when our life is at stake, it is the most important question, because upon the answer hangs the source of our hope and the promise of our recovery.

Joan Borysenko, a renowned scholar and teacher, discovered this in the hospital where she had worked for many years, but she made the discovery as a patient and not as a professional. Driving home from the hospital late one winter night in a state of near exhaustion, she had a head-on collision with another vehicle. She tells us about it in her book *Guilt Is the Teacher, Love Is the Lesson*:

A short time later, near midnight in the early December darkness, the ambulance with flashing lights and shrieking sirens that always carries away some other unfortunate person brought me back to the hospital where I'd worked for so many years. Two orderlies unloaded me into the emergency room, strapped down to a trauma board in case my spinal cord was injured, which, thank God, it was not. Miraculously, the driver of the other car was able to leave the hospital with minor injuries shortly after being examined. Fortunately, I, too, was nearly unscathed, save for one small part of my anatomy. My nose had been literally destroyed—opened like the hood of a car and nearly torn off my face—when my shoulder harness failed to catch.

"How bad is it?" I asked the surgeon as he finished inspecting the damage. "On a scale of one to ten, ten being the worst," I added, in hope of regaining some control, at least in the form of concrete information.

"For you," he replied, "it's a one. You're in no danger and will recover completely. For your nose, it's an eight. I haven't seen anything this bad in years."

My heart sank. "Will it work again? Can you put it back together?"

"I think so. I hope so," he replied, adding, "Do you believe in God?"

I told him that I did. "Well, He was certainly watching out for you tonight. It's a miracle that only your nose was hurt. Why don't you say a prayer?" He then smiled down at me with great kindness, injected the anesthetic, and began the painstaking process of rearranging a nose from its shattered parts.[1]

This was an agonizing experience for Dr. Borysenko, but because she believed in God, she was able to interpret her experience not as a sign of failure but as an act of grace, inviting her to find healing on a deeper level. She acted upon this interpretation, faced her burden of guilt, reordered her priorities, and left one job to create another where she is sharing her faith in a deeper and larger way.

Do you believe in God? If we can answer in the affirmative, then we know that we are not alone, that there is One who cares for us ultimately, with whom we can communicate and who will guide us on our path, even through head-on collisions with disaster.

The character of the God in whom we believe makes all the difference in the world. If the God in whom we believe is a God of love, then we have an ally in our healing. On the other hand, if our God is a God of fear, then we have an enemy. A theological task is, therefore, implicit in our quest for healing. The faith we affirm and how we affirm it is of critical importance to our health.

Affirmation is the process by which we live our faith. The goal of this process is affirmative living, which leads to health and wholeness. Those who seek healing, therefore, must seek affirmative living, which includes awareness, acceptance, action, and affirmation, as well as explicit affirmations of the statements by which we live.[2] We will explore awareness, acceptance, and action later, but let us begin by considering in greater depth how the process of affirmation relates to faith and healing.

FAITH AND HEALING

Affirmative living is literally a matter of life and death, for we grow ill or die when we lack an affirmation strong enough to sustain our lives.

Judith Guest put it this way in her novel *Ordinary People*:

> To have a reason to get up in the morning, it is necessary to possess a guiding principle. A belief of some kind. A bumper sticker, if you will. People in cars on busy freeways call to each other *Boycott Grapes,* comfort each other *Honk If You Love Jesus,* joke with each other *Be Kind to Animals—Kiss a Beaver.* They identify, they summarize, they antagonize with statements of faith.[3]

These words are poignant because they are those of a character named Conrad who lost that guiding principle and tried to take his life. He was found before he could finish the task.

When we lack valid affirmation, our lives seem futile. We are alienated from life, from one another, and from our own selves because we are alienated from God. One of the definitive themes of modernity set forth by Jean-Paul Sartre, Albert Camus, Franz Kafka, Samuel Beckett, and other existentialists has its roots in this futility. Alienated, our hearts become hard. However, it is possible for us to be healed of this hardness of heart by renewing our minds and spirits.

Bernie Siegel, surgeon and Yale professor, tells about Stephanie in his book *Love, Medicine, and Miracles.* Stephanie's doctor diagnosed her cancer and, on a statistical basis, predicted her early death. The doctor said, "All you've got is a hope and a prayer." "How do I hope and pray?" she asked. He answered, "I don't know. It's not my line."[4] Stephanie did learn to hope and to pray through Siegel's Exceptional Cancer Patient program, and she altered the course of her disease and improved her life.

When I first heard Dr. Siegel tell that story, I was touched by Stephanie's plight and by the callousness of the doctor. I wanted to say, "That's my line!" As an ordained Christian minister, finding hope and learning to pray are what I am about. On medical and psychiatric matters, I urge people to seek the best professionals in those fields. But hope and prayer are the specialty of the ministry.

Research is showing that every person must accept a large share of responsibility for his or her health, including prevention as well as recovery from disease and disability. It is important to distinguish between responsibility *in* illness and responsibility *for* illness. Sometimes people do not make this distinction and it adds to their suffering. If a person feels responsible for cancer, this may deepen that person's guilt and add to her or his pain. In many if not most cases, we do not actually know who or what is responsible for an illness. But responsibility in one's illness means that one exercises the ability to respond to whatever the health problem may be in a creative way. We are not passive hosts to illness but active recruiting agents for our well-being. We seek the best medical help we can find, but we are not simply patients to be treated by physicians, nurses, counselors, and other specialists. We are partners with them, and this partnership is to be actively developed from both sides. Moreover, faith, hope, and love—all positive emotions—are also major factors in our healing.

The awareness that faith and healing are related is not new, but the scientific development of the relationship is. The current scientific study stresses verifiability and reproducibility. Much of this research is summed up by Norman Cousins, who was both an explorer and a map maker of this contemporary terrain. The explorer aspects are most evident in his *Anatomy of an Illness* and *The Healing Heart*, in which he described his own illnesses and recoveries. The map maker aspect is most evident in *Head First*, in which he charted the larger territory of medical research.

Of all of Cousins's claims, perhaps the most controversial is that laughter has curative powers. Lying in pain on a hospital bed, Cousins got hold of a projector and some old Marx Brothers films. He made the joyous discovery that ten minutes of belly laughter had an anesthetic effect that would give him two hours of pain-free sleep.

Joey Adams, author and comedian, was "prescribed" to Cousins by his doctor, who wrote on a prescription slip, "Take a Joey Adams story before and after medication." Joey is himself a firm believer that a dose of joy is a spiritual cure. His book *Live Longer Through Laughter* documents this claim. In the foreword to this book, Cousins writes: "Laughter— along with hope, faith, love, will to live, creativity—can be regarded as an important resource in any strategy of recovery or, indeed, in prompting good health."[5]

Joey's use of humor and healing is based on his own experience. His sister tells how, when he was a boy, he would take the family first-aid kit and keep it under his bed. When someone needed a bandage or some iodine, they had to come to "Dr. Adams." Although the healing instinct came early, it was his wife, Cindy, who showed him it could work for him.

Cindy and Joey Adams were making a goodwill tour for the government a few years ago in Southeast Asia. They were in a group of entertainers who were performing for not only the troops but also many of the people of those underdeveloped nations. Eventually the performers stopped entertaining. They began to share their bitterness, their unhappiness, and their discontent, and they were snapping at one another.

Before long, Cindy developed an ear problem. She lost hearing first in one ear and then in the other. It was a serious problem. She went to the doctor, who said, "The only way you're going to solve this is by an operation. We'll have to puncture the ear a bit, create a kind of window which can let some of the sound through. But there's no hope for your hearing apart from that."

Then she went to a primitive doctor in the country. Intuitively, this little woman pierced into the heart of the dilemma, and she communicated to Cindy these words, "Don't hear people; hear God."

She was saying, "Cindy, you're listening to too much negativism and complaint and criticism; and it's making you sick. Stop it! Don't listen to people; listen to God." Cindy began to follow that advice and put away this negativism, complaining, and constant lament and criticism. She began to listen to God, to what God was saying about the opportunity to show love and to be loved.

Soon the hearing came back in one ear and then in the other, and she was cured. "Don't hear people; hear God" is an affirmation that helped both Cindy and Joey.

What the comedian calls one liners, the believer calls affirmations. Both have healing power. Affirmations are God's one liners.

The controversy around humor and healing helped to underscore one of Cousins's major points: Laughter is a metaphor for the positive emotions that contribute to good health. Cousins lived them in defiance of a serious collagen illness and experts' gloomy predictions that he did not have much chance of outliving it. He affirmed his will to live, and he not only recovered but also was regenerated. What marks his recovery from a later heart attack is that the same approach and techniques that had worked before worked again. Reproducibility is one of the acid tests of science, and Cousins had passed it. In *Head First,* Cousins sets his personal experience in the context of vast medical research and documents how "belief became biology."

Alexander Lowen contributed significantly to this discussion most recently in his book *The Spirituality of the Body.* The more Dr. Lowen has explored grace as a function of the body, the more he has discovered grace as a spiritual reality. He writes: "Grace is a state of holiness, of wholeness, of connection to life, and of unity with the divine. This state is also one of health."[6]

Herbert Benson, of Boston's Beth Israel Hospital and the Harvard Medical School, recorded the conclusions of his scientific observations in the United States, the Indian Himalayas, and elsewhere in his books *The Relaxation Response* and *The Mind/Body Effect.* Dr. Benson concluded that there is what he called the relaxation response. He found that certain meditative and prayerful instructions can be employed to lower the heart rate and blood pressure, to decrease the rate of breathing, to slow brain waves, and to bring an overall reduction of the speed of the metabolism. In this relatively peaceful condition, the individual's mental patterns change to counteract the harmful effects and uncomfortable feelings of stress.

Dr. Benson continued his research because, although the relaxation response was helpful, there was something missing. In his further research, Benson found the missing link, which he called the "Faith Factor." The Faith Factor is "a person's deepest personal beliefs combined with the relaxation response."[7] Benson makes these bold claims:

My research and that of others has disclosed that those who develop and use the Faith Factor effectively can: relieve headaches; reduce angina pectoris pains and perhaps even eliminate the need for bypass surgery (an estimated 80 percent of angina pain can be relieved by positive belief!); reduce blood pressure and help control hypertension problems; enhance creativity, especially when experiencing some sort of "mental block"; overcome insomnia; prevent hyperventilation attacks; help alleviate backaches; enhance the therapy of cancer; control panic attacks; lower cholesterol levels; alleviate the symptoms of anxiety that include nausea, vomiting, diarrhea, constipation, short temper, and inability to get along with others; reduce overall stress and achieve greater inner peace and emotional balance.[8]

Dr. Benson outlines the steps by which we can put the Faith Factor to work for us:

1. Pick a focus word or phrase that is rooted in your personal belief system.
2. Choose a comfortable position.
3. Close your eyes.
4. Relax your muscles.
5. Become aware of your breathing, and start using your faith-rooted focus word and breathe very slowly and naturally. Simultaneously repeat your focus word or phrase as you exhale. Use one word or phrase during your sessions so that you'll automatically come to associate it with the calming impact of the Relaxation Response.
6. Assume a passive attitude, and if other thoughts intrude in your mind, gently disregard them.
7. Continue for ten to twenty minutes.
8. Practice the technique twice daily.[9]

With the faith factor, Dr. Benson has provided us with the factor that can contribute to our wellness, but we must provide the faith.

AFFIRMATIONS

Affirmations are explicit statements of faith that may be used within a healing context. Affirmations function as the "focus word or phrase which is rooted in your personal belief system."

There are basically two ways to use affirmations in the process that Dr. Benson calls the faith factor. One way is to begin with a statement of faith drawn from the Bible or a creed or another witness of the faith. The other way is to draw directly on our personal resources. Here are some examples of the first way.

Affirmations of the Creator: "My God is granting me life as a gift now." Think this as you inhale, and as you exhale, think, "I am offering my life as a gift now." Another affirmation: "Divine love is creating through me now."

Affirmations of the Redeemer: "Lord, I do love you." "Lord, I trust my life to you." "Loving is living for me." "Lord Jesus Christ, have mercy on me." This is the "Jesus Prayer" made famous through the classic *The Way of the Pilgrim.* Biblical verses also may be paraphrased, such as "I can do all things through Christ who strengthens me" (Phil. 4:13).

Affirmations of the Holy Spirit: "Come, Holy Spirit, come." "I am receiving your comfort now, Lord." "I am a child of the dawn."

No affirmation is limited to any one season, and some are especially durable, such as "Lord, thy will, not mine, be done" and "Letting go of it all now, I am walking humbly with you, Lord."

We also may draw directly on our personal resources for affirmations. The following step-by-step process can help us to find our own personal affirmation, which is rooted in our belief system. It is adapted from *Into the Light,* by Ron Delbene with Mary and Herb Montgomery:

Step 1. First, pick a focus word or phrase that is rooted in your own personal belief system.

• What is the name for God that is most meaningful for you? Think about it a moment and write it down (a 3" x 5" card is effective). Is the word *God?* Is it *Our heavenly Father? Lord?* Whatever is your favorite name for God, write that down.

• What do you most want in your life right now? Is it peace, love, joy? Whatever it is, write that down. I know that this is dangerous, because what you most want may not be what you most need in your life right now. You may want money when what you need most deeply is faith. Nevertheless, write down what you want most deeply at this point in your life, whatever it is.

• Write a sentence in which God, called by your favorite name, is granting you the thing you most deeply need. For example: "My Father in heaven is granting me peace of mind"; or "God is granting me the way to resolve conflict"; or "God is ending my family's turmoil"; or "God Almighty is granting me health and happiness."

This is your affirmation. This is your theology in its basic personal form and open to revision. You're saying that this is what you truly believe at the moment, what you in fact live by. This is the key to your personal belief system to be developed by experience, reason, scripture, and tradition. This is your affirmation. This is your Faith Factor.

Step 2. Choose a comfortable position. There are many positions, some with crossed legs, but for us it is perfectly acceptable simply to sit in a chair with feet firmly on the floor and hands held together or placed just above the knees. Just be comfortable.

Step 3. Close your eyes. Don't squeeze them shut or squint; just close them naturally.

Step 4. Relax your muscles, starting at the feet and progressing up through your calves, thighs, and abdomen. Loosen up your head, neck, and shoulders by gently turning your head from side to side and shrugging your shoulders slightly. Stretch and relax your arms and hands; let them drape naturally in your lap. Don't grasp your knees or legs or hold your hands tightly together.

Step 5. Breathe naturally and slowly; don't force the rhythm. Start to repeat your affirmation silently. For example, slowly breathe in and out, and as your breath is going out, say, "My Lord is granting me peace now." Breathe in silently and then, while you're breathing out, repeat your affirmation. Continue to do this as you breathe in and out.

Step 6. Maintain a passive attitude. Sit quietly, repeating your affirmation. You will find that other thoughts begin to invade your mind. That is all right; just let them come and go. Come back again to your affirmation and repeat it.

Step 7. Continue this for ten to twenty minutes.

Step 8. Practice the method twice daily; before breakfast and dinner are times many people find appropriate.[10]

These are some examples of affirmations that express the faith of the Christian community across the centuries as well as our personal faith. They are expressions of the ground of our hope and the power of our prayer. Such a beginning may seem small and insignificant, but it is like the mustard seed, which is barely visible at first but grows into a mighty and productive tree. Similarly, as we live these affirmations, we discover that what begins in our personal experience may grow to embrace a wider range of faith.

In addition to a personal affirmation, there are affirmations that are expressive of the fundamental principles of our faith. These grow out of our experience and response to the Bible. The Trinity, for example, is incorporated in our lives by affirmation.

NEGATION

Now we must deal with the dark side of affirmation: negation. There is a popular view that affirmation is a bright and breezy approach in which just by thinking positively and repeating phrases to ourselves wonderful things will simply materialize, and we will live happily ever after. There are some whose work may lead to this view, but I believe it to be not only untrue but also dangerous.

Genuine affirmation is not only countered by negation, but it also actually stirs it up. If we are not prepared for this, we can be in deep trouble. Lisa, who is serious in her affirmation, likens her experience to pushing a plunger into the toilet. The push is a positive thrust, but it will bring forth something foul and ugly. Affirmation, like the plunger, will bring forth what runs counter to our view of the good life, but if we honestly deal with that, we can flush ourselves of waste and be cleansed.

This is not easy. The shock that comes when we first encounter the negatives may be overwhelming. It may cause mental, emotional, and spiritual disturbance. We may be so repelled by what comes up that we abandon the whole affirmation process right there.

In truth, this conflict is a sign that the affirmation is beginning to work. We are passing from faith as fantasy to faith as reality. Only by facing what arises at this point and dealing with it can affirmation be authentic—that is, genuine and effective. This is when we discover the truth of the words, "Do not be overcome by evil, but overcome evil with good" (Rom. 12:21).

There are many different ways of accounting for this phenomenon, and we will consider some of them later. But the point is that in dealing with the negations, we find depth and fullness that we lacked, and we move toward wholeness and healing.

Now let us focus on how to deal with the issue of negativity in practice. I have found that it is most effective to write our affirmations. This is not strictly necessary, and at times it is not possible. But for maximum effectiveness, the affirmations should be written and developed as part of one's journal.[11]

While you are focusing on the affirmation, write it down. Then write down your reaction.

Come back to your breathing, then write the affirmation again. Then the reaction. Then the affirmation, and so on. Then look at what is happening. Perhaps the best way to describe this process is to quote from my own journal. In this example from my journal, the originating voice is italicized, the reaction is not.

My God is granting me peace and joy.
But I do not feel peaceful or joyful.
My God is granting me peace and joy.
But I feel anxious and sad.
(Adjustment: God is granting me peace and joy, but I am not receiving it. Therefore)
I am receiving God's peace and joy.
Ah! Receiving God's peace and joy.
God's peace and joy are washing over me.
God's peace is flowing into me. (Here affirmation and reaction join.)
I visualize peace like a warm, golden light slowly flowing over me, pushing darkness and sluggishness down, down. Peace flowing over me. Peace flowing over my head, face, shoulders, arms, trunk, bottom, legs, feet. All of me.
Peace.
Peace. (Now this one word carries the affirmation.)
Peace—breathing in peace.
Peace—breathing out peace.
Peace. Peace. Peace.

Gradually I am filled with this peace and carry it into my work for the day. It is typical in my experience for affirmations to work in this dialectical way, with negation and with simplification, visualization, deepened breathing, and energizing for action. (For more discussion of visualization and its role in healing, see Kenneth R. Pelletier's *Mind as Healer, Mind as Slayer: A Holistic Approach to Preventing Stress Disor-*

ders. See also *Getting Well Again* by Dr. O. Carl Simonton, Stephanie Matthews-Simonton, and James Creigton; as well as Shakti Gawain's *Creative Visualization*.)

What we tend to discover if we stay with this process is that we are led past repetition and reaction deeper and deeper into our own spirit and the Holy Spirit until it is as if we are not making the affirmation but the affirmation is making us.

AFFIRMATIVE LIVING

Affirmations are a vital instrument for affirmative living, but affirmations must be taken up into our life-style. We cannot simply repeat words and expect change. Affirmative living also calls for awareness, acceptance, action, and the process of affirmation. We touched upon these processes briefly in the previous chapter, but here we will explore each in greater detail.

Awareness means paying attention to what is going on within as well as around us. This sounds simple, but sadly it is a rare achievement. It is a truism that many people today walk around like zombies. Many people not only "sleepwalk" through each day, unaware of the social and political activities around them, but they also sleepwalk through their own lives, not really tuned in to what is going on within them—what they really feel, think, or deeply need and desire in their brief stay here on earth. They are not really present to their own lives.

One obvious example of our not being tuned in to our lives is our breathing—a basic function and sign of human life. The inspiration of the spirit is directly related to the respiration of the body, and this relationship is a key to health, and that fact is becoming increasingly recognized (see *The Miracle of Mindfulness: A Manual on Meditation* by Thich Nhat Hanh; *Full Catastrophe Living: Using the Wisdom of Your Body to Face Stress,*

Pain and Illness by Jon Kabat-Zinn; and *The Meditative Mind* by Daniel Goleman). Few people are aware of their breathing and how dangerously shallow it is.

One evening, as I was about to lead an affirmation group in a breathing exercise, a young woman who is a dancer by profession, cried out, "Wait! Before you move, pay attention to how you are breathing and how you are holding yourself right now." We did this, and we were shocked. We had thought of ourselves, no doubt, as being relatively at ease, sitting on comfortable chairs or sofas. But when we stopped to look carefully at ourselves, we were shocked to see how tightly our bodies were tied up, how tense we were, and how shallow our breathing was.

Breathing for all of us was light and for most confined to the head, the nasal passages. Most of us had probably been breathing at that level throughout the day, neither using nor developing our capacity for deeper breathing—allowing the breath more fully into the lungs and deeper into the body— which would have given us more energy and aliveness. We were able to move toward that deeper breathing, but first we had to be aware.

Acceptance means admitting that our situation is what it is, whether we like it or not. Acceptance does not mean that we condone the situation, but simply that we recognize it for what it is rather than the way we wish it were. Freud said that the wish that things were different is the root of neurosis. Denial that we are where we are rather than where we wish to be is a common enemy.

A young woman named Wilma came to a therapist with her mother. The therapist asked what it was that brought the young woman to him. "It's awful," Wilma blurted out, "but people are always calling me fat."

"It's awful," chimed in the mother. "Everywhere she goes, people tell her she's fat. They make fun of her. People are so cruel. What can we do?"

The therapist turned to the young woman and said, "Let's face it, Wilma, you're fat!"

At this the young woman burst into tears, and the mother practically leaped from her seat. But when the weeping and wailing had run their course, daughter and mother had to face the obvious. People said that Wilma was fat because Wilma was fat. She had to accept the fact that she was overweight if she were going to deal with her situation. Denying it and blaming others would get her nowhere.

Action means doing what needs to be done to deal with our situation. We cannot sit passively by and wait for things to improve. We must do what we can to move us toward our vision, however small that action may be. Once we take that step, our energy tends to increase. This is crucial. Much of what happens to us is beyond our control, but we can decide how we are going to respond. We can be proactive, taking steps in advance to prevent dire straits and create better lives.

Wilma, for example, not only came to accept the obesity of which others had made her aware, but she took action to end it as well. She went on a diet, exercised, and became slimmer and healthier. But that came only after her action.

A person has room to act even in the most difficult circumstances. Mickey and Pat have been deeply involved with Pop Henry, Mickey's stepfather. Pop Henry, eighty years old, lost both legs because of a car accident. Instead of becoming bitter, he was a continuing inspiration to family, doctors, and nurses, and was soon planning to resume swimming and other activities he enjoyed. He was eager to get his prosthesis and be "on his feet again." This man is a vivid example of how people can take steps toward wholeness, even when they have no legs.

Affirmation (the *process*) means that we cheer God and ourselves no matter how things are going at a given moment. Our ultimate value is based on the love of God and not how we are feeling at a certain point in time.

Wilma can affirm herself as a person of sacred worth even while she is overweight. Pop Henry is loved even without his legs and his former physical prowess. You can affirm yourself as loved, supported, and inspired by God, even in the moment of your greatest defeat or deepest despair. In fact, affirmation is fundamental to the whole process of affirmative living; it underlies it and grows out of it.

There is a spiraling effect in the process of affirmative living. Awareness gives rise to acceptance, which gives rise to action, which gives rise to affirmation, which gives rise to greater awareness, and so forth. This process may extend over longer periods of time. Thus periods of our life—days or weeks—may be characterized by one of these elements. We may have a season of awareness, or it may take us several seasons to gain acceptance.

The process of affirmative living can also be used as a guide to meditation. That is, on a regular basis, we may choose to examine our lives, to become aware, to accept what we find, to choose the action most appropriate, and to affirm ourselves and God.

Affirmative living also works as a healing method. In a time of crisis or pain, we can become aware: Where do we hurt? What is going on? We can accept ourselves and our situation whether we like it or not. We can settle on the action that is best to take. And we can affirm God and ourselves in the process.

In all these ways our explicit affirmations, the statements we have discovered or created, carry the affirmative spirit. And in all these ways the affirmations are ingredients in and expressive of affirmative living.

Let me give one example: A young man named Bill was engaged to be married. In fact, he was just about to be married when his fiancée decided she did not want to go through with the wedding. Bill was in a state of shock. He loved this woman very deeply and had no idea of how he could even

43

live without her. The break was totally unexpected. It was all he could do to make his way back to his room.

Bill was a believer, and this was a great test of his faith, but he affirmed that God would help him through this crisis, and he earnestly prayed that this would be the case. It dawned on him that he must forgive this woman for acting in a way that was so devastating to him. He prayed that he could forgive her, and then he realized that there were many others he needed to forgive. There was a time of weeping and cleansing as he went through his life and sought to find the grace to forgive all who had hurt him. Then he realized he had to find forgiveness from all the people whom he had hurt. Throughout all this he believed that God was granting this forgiveness; he actually experienced that forgiveness.

Bill described a moment in which he could actually feel God's presence in the room. It was when his heart was breaking with an enormous pain. Suddenly it seemed as if God were a mighty force descending palpably into the room from above. And this great, warm power descended upon him and took the enormous pain and crushed it down until it was small. It was as if some kind of spiritual compactor had entered the room and crushed his great pain into a small ball. And then this Presence lifted and went up out of the room.

Bill said he still felt the pain, but because of the Presence that pain had been overcome. It was smaller now. He could deal with it; he could go on with his life. He had found hope and prayer.

If you want to enjoy the benefits of affirmation, take it up into your life, as Søren Kierkegaard counseled, and practiced it regularly.

God is a God of love, loving us through creation, redemption, and sustenance: the Holy Trinity. Yet, to recover the healing power of the Trinity, we must sort through the wreckage of our time.

CHAPTER
THREE

TRINITY

The Power of Love

THE TRINITY: HOLY AND UNHOLY

J. Robert Oppenheimer, the scientist known as the father of the atomic bomb, was reading a book of John Donne's poems in 1944 when the word came that a site had been chosen for the bomb's first test. The caller urged that a code name for the site be fixed immediately. Oppenheimer turned to the opening lines of the sonnet he had just read:

Batter my heart, three-personed God, for you
As yet but knock, breathe, shine and seek.[1]

"Trinity," Oppenheimer said softly. "We'll call it Trinity."[2] Thus was the most destructive force in human history given the name of the Christian God of creative love.

At Trinity on a night in July 1945, the first atomic explosion went off. In his book *Day of Trinity*, Lansing Lamont writes:

No living thing touched by that raging furnace survived. Within a millisecond the fireball had struck the ground, flattening out its base and acquiring a skirt of molten black dust that boiled and billowed in all directions. Within twenty-five milliseconds the fireball had expanded to a point where the Washington Monument would have been enveloped. At

45

8/10th's of a second the ball's white hot dome had topped the Empire State Building. The shock wave caromed across the rolling desert. . . . The stench of death clung to the desert in the vicinity of the detonation. No rattlesnake or lizard, nothing that could crawl or fly was left. The Yuccas and Joshua trees had disappeared in the heat storm. No solitary blade of grass was visible.[3]

Trinity. We'll call it Trinity. The test at Trinity was soon followed by the actual use of the bomb in war. On August 6, 1945, the atomic bomb was dropped on Hiroshima, Japan, and blew three-fifths of the city off the face of the earth.

Before Oppenheimer announced what had happened to his colleagues in the Los Alamos auditorium, he clasped his hands above his head like a prize fighter signaling victory; then he told them about the atomic bomb that had killed seventy-eight thousand men, women, and children and left thousands of others to a slow and painful death. Trinity. We'll call it Trinity.

And today we have bombs so much more powerful and systems for delivering them so much more sophisticated that they make the mushroom cloud of Hiroshima look like a toadstool—the devastation almost trivial by comparison. And we have them in enormous quantities.

Trinity—the destructive force that is both effected and symbolized by bombs? No thank you, Dr. Oppenheimer. We will call *this* Trinity, the Trinity of the Bible, the God of powerful love.

We must learn to live by the power of love or we shall die by the love of power. Make no mistake; there is power in love: the power to create and recreate, the power to form and to transform. It is the power of which John Donne spoke in his poem as "Your force to break, blow, burn and make me new."

The power of love is the power of compassion, dialogue, reasoning, sharing, and persuasion. It is not the power of vindictiveness, monologue, irrationality, and coercion. Both the Old and the New Testaments reveal a God who expresses power in love.

The God of the Old Testament is full of power, but as Nehemiah put it, this is power that redeems (Neh. 1:10). The characteristic New Testament word for power is *dynamis*, from which we get our word *dynamite*. So Paul writes in Romans 1:17, "The one who is righteous will live by faith."

Faith is the activity by which the power of God is received personally and transmuted into power for living. By faith we come "on line" so the love of God flows through us to others. New life begins for anyone.

Salvation by grace through faith means that God triumphs over every obstacle between God and humanity, except human freedom. Justification means that human love removes that last obstacle. In our freedom we choose to love as God loves us. The power of God is the saving power of love.

The power of God also sustains us. The Holy Spirit, often symbolized by fire, is like the slow burning conflagration that carries capsules into outer space and brings them back again. The love of God is known to us not only in the creation of the world and the redemption of humanity but also in our day-to-day existence amid the dramas of personal and interrelational life. God sustains and guides us through the Holy Spirit.

By powerful love, God creates the world. By powerful love, God blasts away the sin that has come between the Creator and the creation. By powerful love, God sustains life.

What it comes down to is whether we shall live by the Trinity of the Bible or die by the Trinity of the bomb. Are we to be bombers or believers? If we are to be believers, we must mobilize an understanding of the Holy Trinity that is grounded in the power of love.

God cares for all creatures (Psalm 104), protects all that lives (Genesis 9), creates ecological spaces where life is possible (Genesis 1), and initiates relationships between different kinds of living beings for their mutual enrichment. God is turned toward the whole creation in love.

Jesus Christ is the incarnation of this suffering love. In his life, death, and resurrection, God empties the divine Self of glory and becomes poor and vulnerable for our sake (Phil. 2:5-9). Thus God's ownership of the world is defined by the pathos of love—by parental yearning for and suffering with the whole creation (Romans 8).

Our hope, therefore, as we consider the plight of a groaning creation isgrounded in God's sovereignty and the sovereignty of God's love, over which no threat of death or decay can have ultimate sway.

At times we grow weary and may despair because there seems to be so few who worship the Holy Trinity and so many who worship destruction. It helps to know that even amid the bombing of Japan there were believers. One of them was Kiyoshi Tanimoto, pastor of the Methodist Church of Hiroshima. On the morning of August 6, 1945, he had gotten up early to help a parishioner who had helped him the day before. He rested a while from pushing a heavy handcart. The morning was pleasant. Suddenly a tremendous flash of light cut the sky. Tanimoto and his friend had time to react with horror since they were about two miles from the center of the explosion. When Tanimoto looked up after being showered with fragments of wood and tile, he saw that the house next to him had collapsed. Clouds of dust had arisen to form an eerie twilight.

"I've got to get out of here," he thought, and he started to run, not even thinking about his friend. As he ran he saw ruins, people coming out of them with blood running from their heads, chests, and backs. He saw one elderly woman walking along in a daze carrying a little boy on her back. Suddenly Tanimoto became aware. He asked himself, "Why am I running? I am a Methodist minister. I should not be running, I should be helping people." He stopped running and walked over to the woman, who was crying, "I'm hurt!

I'm hurt!" Tanimoto took the child from her back and put it on his own. He took the woman by the hand and led her to an emergency shelter. In that act, Tanimoto's terror left him.[4]

By caring for the old woman and young boy, he was lifted out of his self-absorption and into concern for others, which led him to countless acts of service. He went back to help his friend who had fallen. And once more he ran. But this time he ran not in fear but to help by seeking medical care, offering support and comfort, and finding ways of rebuilding. Tanimoto gave the remaining years of his active ministry to the recovery of the people of Hiroshima and the healing of wounds, including involvement with Norman Cousins in treatment of the Hiroshima maidens. He was a believer, not a bomber.

THE TRINITY AND THE BIBLE

When John Donne wrote of the three-personed God, whose name was later taken in vain by the creators of the atomic bomb, he gave voice to a reality that underlies faith from the beginning of creation, revealed through Christ and the Bible, and that sustains the church through the ages.

The Bible is fundamentally trinitarian in its message. Specific passages refer to the threefold nature of God, but they are expressions of this thoroughgoing affirmation rather than proof of it. For example, in 1 Corinthians 12:4-6, Paul correlates Spirit, Lord, and God (see also Eph. 4:4-6 and 2 Cor. 13:14). In the Old Testament the concepts of the Spirit and Wisdom of God (see Prov. 8.22ff.) influenced a number of New Testament passages that became foundations for the later formulation of doctrine (see John 1:15ff.; Col. 1:15ff.; Heb. 1:2-3). Many passages relate to this theme.

F. F. Bruce was a biblical scholar who considered the texts cited above and wrote of the Trinity: "The coexistence of Father, Son and Holy Spirit in the Unity of the Godhead;

while not a biblical term, 'Trinity' represents the crystal-lization of New Testament teaching."[5]

THE TRINITY IN HISTORY

How the God who is revealed in the Bible is to be under-stood as Father, Son, and Holy Spirit has been a study of immense importance from the early days of the church. The term *Trinity,* from the Latin *Trinitas,* seems to have been used first by Tertullian, while the Greek term *trias,* which corre-sponds to it, apparently was used first by Theophilus, his older contemporary.

The Trinity proclaims one God in three persons. The "threeness" expresses itself in persons who are clearly iden-tifiable in the classical tradition as Father, Son, and Holy Spirit, persons who create, redeem, and support. Most of the attention of the church is paid to the persons and the works of the Trinity, but unless this threeness is grounded in one-ness, faith may veer into unitheism. In other words, one person of the Trinity, Jesus, for instance, is asked to function for the whole. Or faith may veer into polytheism, where in effect we have three gods or other heresies. Therefore, the church has again and again examined its faith and been called back to the affirmation of the unity as well as to the diversity of the Trinity.

There are numerous ways in which this unity may be approached—historical, philosophical, psychological, mys-tical, devotional, existential, relational, and so forth. Histori-cally, it was of critical importance to the first Christians that the God whom they worshiped was none other than the God of Israel. The God who made himself known in Jesus of Nazareth was not a new God but the God of Abraham, Isaac, and Jacob. To be sure, Jesus challenged the understanding of the Jewish establishment of his day ("Moses said unto you, but I say unto you . . . "), but he did so in the name of the God who had revealed himself to Moses. The Shema of Israel

("Hear O Israel, the Lord our God is one") was incorporated into the *schema* of Christianity. This one God is revealed as Creator, Redeemer, and Sustainer. To declare the oneness of God in the three is essential to Christianity's understanding of itself as continuous (as well as discontinuous) from Judaism with an authentic claim of the history of revelation through Israel and the Scriptures. Similar continuities and discontinuities can be found between Christianity and other world religions, but the centrality of love is common to all.

Space does not permit us to pursue the historical development of the Trinity here, but fortunately numerous resources are available for further study.[6]

THE ONE WHO LOVES AS THREE

God is the one who loves as three. I propose this approach to the Trinity because it draws together many differing lines of interpretation at the point where they make an impact on our lives.

The use of love in interpreting the Trinity has dangers because the word is so often sentimentalized and trivialized. The temptation is to discard the word. But as Sam Keen puts it in his book *The Passionate Life: Stages of Loving,* the problem is not so much with our tongues as it is with our hearts. We cannot live the passionate life without a passionate God.

God is love, as John put it, and God loves us in creating, redeeming, and sustaining us. The most appropriate response to this God is for us to love. This is revealed in Jesus' response to the question as to what is the greatest commandment: "You shall love the Lord your God and your neighbor as yourself." The Creator, Redeemer, and Sustainer calls us to love God, neighbor, and self. The triune God calls us to a triune love.

Augustine explored the Trinity from many different angles without denying its mystery. He came to see that love is the key. He wrote in *De Trinitate:*

Behold, then, there are three things: he that loves, and that which is loved, and love. What then is love, except a certain life which couples or seeks to couple together some things, namely him that loves, and that which is loved? And this is so even in outward and carnal loves. . . . What does the mind love in a friend except the mind? There, then, also are three things: he that loves, and that which is loved and love.[7]

David Miller acknowledges that Augustine's metaphor of love and marriage for the Trinity may at first seem farfetched. But Miller goes on to show how common the metaphor is, not only in Hebrew and Greek thought but also in contemporary literature and experience. Miller writes in *Three Faces of God*: "It is an affair from beginning to end, a ménage à trois, a divine menagerie of love. The formula of the Christian doctrine of the Trinity, together with its residual fantasy, brings to expression what we know all too well from life."[8]

Augustine, having established the likeness of the Trinity to human love, went on to point out the unlikeness, as Miller notes. Both sides of Augustine's paradox must be kept before us. The Trinity is like our human love; the Trinity is unlike our human love.

The likeness and unlikeness of the Trinity to our love is akin to our likeness and unlikeness to God. We are like God (made in God's image), but we are not God. Yet love can be a bridge between God and ourselves, between ourselves and others, and even between our divided inner selves.

In the *Bridge of San Luis Rey*, Thornton Wilder tells of the collapse of the finest bridge in Peru in which five people plunge to their deaths. Dona Clara ponders the tragedy as she works with the sick and the blind in the hospital. She concludes:

But soon we shall die and all memory of those five will have left the earth, and we ourselves shall be loved for a while and forgotten. But the love will have been enough; all those impulses of love return to the love that made them. Even memory is not necessary for love. There is a land of the living and a land of the dead, and the bridge is love, the only survival, the only meaning.[9]

The bridge of love is created, redeemed, and sustained by God.

C H A P T E R
F O U R

GOD'S LOVE CREATES:
Care for Our Health and Care for the Earth

The innate capacity for healing which is essential to our recovery is given to us by our Creator, according to Bernie S. Siegel and many others. What makes Siegel's claim authoritative is that he is a medical doctor, a surgeon, who bases his claim on his experience with cancer patients. In *Peace, Love, and Healing,* he writes: "Our Creator has given us five senses to help us survive threats from the external world, and a sixth sense, our healing system, to help us survive internal threats."[1]

Love is also integral to healing because it links the divine and the human physiologically. Siegel refers to David C. McClelland, a Harvard professor who is engaged in research on what he calls "the love variables" and their impact on the endocrine system. These variables are self-love and divine love, the latter referring to that noninvolved action that he finds in many religiously inspired people. Such people are not worried about their egos. They are not concerned about whether they are succeeding or failing. They act from the heart.

Siegel also cites Evy McDonald as living proof of the relation of self-love and divine love to healing. When she was diagnosed with amyotrophic lateral sclerosis (ALS, known as Lou Gehrig's disease) in 1980, she was told by her neurologist that she had only six months to live, and that if she wanted to do something nice, she should leave her body to science. That same afternoon she was fired from her job as a nurse because she had been out sick so much; that evening she discovered that her apartment had been burglarized and all her valuables had been stolen.

McDonald might have found the doctor's advice tempting at that point, but she decided on a different course. She knew that death was inevitable, but she had a strong compulsion to discover what unconditional love was before she died. She also knew that her first step toward self-love would mean acceptance of her body, which she had always hated and which was now wasted and deteriorating. McDonald began to notice and write down how many negative and positive thoughts she had about her body throughout the day. When she saw the preponderance of negative thoughts, she had to confront the hatred she had for her body.

McDonald countered this habitual hatred by singling out every day one aspect of her physical body, no matter how small, that was acceptable to her. Then she would use that item to rewrite her negative list, following every negative thought with a positive one, such as "My hair is truly pretty" or "I have lovely hands."

As each day a different positive item was added to the rewriting, she felt like a jigsaw puzzle being put back together. When the last piece fell into place, her mind shifted, and she saw the whole picture: It was perfect. The body she saw in the mirror was, in her words, "a bowl of jelly in a wheelchair," but for the first time in her life she knew her body to be aesthetically pleasing. Her "complete, unalterable acceptance" of the way her body was brought her total peace.

Moreover, her physical body stopped deteriorating. This reversal was a by-product of all the other changes. McDonald said, "Physical healing did not occur because I set out to 'cure' myself, but because my job on earth was not complete. . . . Since then I joyously awake each day, filled with enthusiasm, and continue to play my role in the transformation of medical practice." McDonald had come to accept her illness as a challenge and a gift and was positively transformed by it.

Siegel points out that McDonald's goal "was to discover the experience of unconditional love, not to avoid dying. She was not setting herself up for failure, but for an experience that was within her power to give herself. Love and healing are always possible, even when a cure is not."[2]

Many theological challenges and gifts are packed within this account and others like it. We may pass over them quickly or even dismiss them, but if we consider them seriously, we shall be led to powerful resources for transformation and healing.

THE CREATOR GOD AND THE CREATION STORY

The biblical story of creation in the book of Genesis offers powerful resources for health and healing. Briefly put, those include these views:

- We live in a cosmos rather than a chaos because the Creator God is like a loving parent who intends our good.
- Creation is purposeful, and wellness is intended.
- Sexuality is a part of God's good creation and of good health.
- Humans are creative creatures, capable of choice. God intends creation, but humans may choose destruction.
- Creation is a continuing activity in which we all participate. Care for the earth is essential for our health.
- Humans have chosen ways other than God's, and therefore creation calls for redemption.

This Creator who gives us our innate capacity to heal is God, who, according to the Christian faith, can be approached as a loving parent. The Apostles' Creed, regarded as definitive for all Christians, begins: "I believe in God, the

Father Almighty, Maker of heaven and earth." The basis of this creed is the Bible and the early church's interpretation of it. Although the biblical story of the Garden of Eden is allegorical, it is nevertheless reenacted symbolically in our own lives, as Alexander Lowen points out. We will now explore the Creation story and some of its aftermath, drawing out implications for health and healing.

The biblical story of creation is a statement of faith, but so are all creation stories. The biblical story presents a story of faith in a personal Being whose intention is to create a good space out of a formless void. It is richly poetic and contrasts with the databased speculations of some scientific theories. The image of God shaping dust into human form and breathing life into it may seem too simple for today's sophisticate, but the dignity of humanity and the self-esteem of individuals rest on the faith that we are made in the image of God. The Bible begins with this theme. The first words are, "In the beginning when God created the heavens and the earth, the earth was a formless void and darkness covered the face of the deep, while a wind from God swept over the face of the waters. Then God said, 'Let there be light'; and there was light. And God saw that the light was good; and God separated the light from the darkness" (Gen. 1:1-4).

The book of Genesis proceeds to show how God continues to create out of the original chaos an orderly world of night and day, earth and sea, vegetation and living creatures. Having brought this ordered world into being, God creates humankind in "our image," male and female. God blesses them and bids them be fruitful and multiply and have dominion over the plants and animals (Gen. 1:27-30).

A further account from another tradition shows the Lord forming man from the dust of the ground and breathing into his nostrils the breath of life, and the man becomes a living being. In this story as well man is commanded to take care of the garden, but the Lord observes that it is not good for the man to be alone, so the Lord puts Adam into a deep sleep and creates from his rib a woman.

Then the man said,
"This at last is bone of my bones
and flesh of my flesh;
this one shall be called Woman,
for out of Man this one was taken."
Therefore a man leaves his father and his mother and clings to his wife, and they become one flesh. And the man and his wife were both naked, and were not ashamed. (Gen. 2:23-25)

Sex is regarded as a God-given impulse, drawing a man and a woman together that they may become one flesh. This has God's blessing and is not regarded as evil. The man and the woman are both naked, and they are not ashamed.

Adam and Eve, the archetypal man and woman, are placed by God in the Garden of Eden, the archetypal paradise, and are commanded to take care of it. They may freely eat of every tree of the garden except one, the tree of the knowledge of good and evil. Should they eat of that fruit, that will be the day that they die.

The serpent appears, who is craftier than any other animal. He engages in an elaborate conversation with Eve, claiming that she will not surely die if she eats the forbidden fruit but instead "will be like God, knowing good and evil." Eve looks again at the tree and, perceiving that its fruit is good food and that it will make her wise, she eats and persuades Adam to eat as well. Suddenly they become aware that they are naked. They are so ashamed that they sew leaves together to cover themselves.

God appears in the garden, and Adam and Eve try to hide. "Adam, where are you?" God calls. Adam responds that he is hiding because he is naked. Adam tries to pin the blame for their newfound knowledge on Eve, who in turn blames the serpent. The serpent, the woman, and the man are progressively called to account. The serpent henceforth will be cursed to crawl upon the earth. Eve will henceforth experience pain in childbirth, and Adam will toil all his days. Adam and Eve are then expelled from the Garden of Eden by the Lord God, who reasons that since they have eaten of the tree of the knowledge of good and evil, they might also reach out for the tree of life and become immortal. The way back to the garden and the tree of life is barred by an angel with a flaming sword.

The way forward includes the first murder—Cain's slaying of his brother Abel (Genesis 4)—the flood and God's covenant with Noah to preserve the earth (Genesis 6–10); the formation of Israel as a community of faith and a nation (Genesis 12–50); and the captivity of Israel in Egypt, the emergence of Moses, and the giving of the Law (Exodus).

THE CHARACTER OF THE CREATOR

To fully understand God as Creator and the implications of this for healing, it is helpful to further explore the character of God. The act of creation is at once passionate and compassionate. The Creator brings the world into being not out of necessity but out of a passionate joy. God creates man and then his companion, woman, because God does not want man to be alone. God continues to care for all creation. God is the Supreme Lover.

The Creator Is Like a Faithful Father

To speak of God as Creator and Lover is to draw closer to God as Father. God as Creator is powerful but distant. God as One who creates out of love is closer but possibly unconstant. The God of the Bible is not a cosmic Casanova but a faithful Father. To the question of what God is like, no answer has recurred more than that of the psalmist: "like a father." And not just any kind of father, but a father who loves his children and honors those who love him.

God is referred to as Father in both the Old and the New Testaments, although there are important distinctions between these references. The reference just cited from the Psalms calls God fatherly because he loves and cares for his children. But God is more than a father in the ordinary sense in that he is also "a father to the fatherless" (Ps. 68:5). God goes beyond the bounds of ordinary fatherhood and embraces even orphans as his own.

The New Testament retains this sense of God as a loving father of all his children with two significant additions. First, God is referred to as the Father of Jesus Christ. Jesus understood himself as being identified with God the Father. This was essential to his healing work as he made clear in his healing of the partially paralyzed man at the Pool of Bethesda. When questioned by the religionists as to how he dared to heal on the Sabbath, Jesus replied that his Father was working then and so was he. The healing activity of Jesus Christ cannot be understood as an isolated phenomenon but as part of the ongoing work of the Father. This so infuriated Jesus' opponents that they began to plot his death, for he had not only violated the Sabbath but also claimed to be equal with God (John 5:17-24). The early church accepted Jesus' identity with the Father and made it basic in its creeds and worship.

The New Testament is further distinguished in that God is not only referred to as a father but also is addressed as Father. This is a radical departure from the Old Testament.

God is like a father in that he loves and cares for all his children. Jesus related to God as his father, especially in carrying out his healing ministry, and he taught us to pray to God as "our Father."

The Creator Is More Than a Father

All language about God is metaphorical. To believe otherwise is to create an idol. In calling God "Father," we epitomize God as personal and as providential. But God is more than a father. Donald W. Shriver, Jr., writes helpfully in *The Lord's Prayer: A Way of Life:*

> It is high time that men in church inquired into the spiritual dangers of exclusive preoccupations with male imagery for God. It is high time that all church people, women and men, reappropriated those aspects of Jesus' ministry that make abundantly clear his own break with many a male-supremacy assumption of his society. . . . So whether we are learning to say "Father" with a sense of the rightness of saying "Mother," too, or are learning to say "Mother" without denying that God can use analogies of fatherhood in spite of our misunderstanding of the same, we shall indeed have to be learners, all of us, and all of us teachers, as well.[3]

Across the centuries, feminine images have enriched our understanding of God. These permeate the Bible, as Virginia Ramey Mollenkott has pointed out:

> *Hosea 13:8* depicts God turning in anger against wickedness like a mother bear bereaved of her whelps. *Deuteronomy 32:11-12* depicts God as a mother eagle stirring up her nest full of eaglets, teaching them to fly on their own. *Isaiah 42:14* depicts God as a woman in labor, and *Isaiah 49:15*, as a lactating woman unable to forget the offspring that she suckles tenderly at her breast. *Psalm 123:2* pictures God as the head woman in a household, to whom humanity looks just as the maidens look to their mistress for guidance.[4]

Our understanding of the nature of God is enriched by associating with the divine elements that we tend to think of as feminine: mother, sister, nurture, compassion, tenderness, and mystery. To refer to God as mother as well as father is a dramatic way of expressing a new consciousness. However, the female aspect of the divine must not be restricted to the father-mother metaphor. The values of the feminine are at work also in incarnation, redemption, and the Holy Spirit. To acknowledge the feminine aspects of the divine calls for a corresponding recognition of the status and role of women throughout history and in our current situation.

We see this agenda in *Beyond God the Father* by Mary Daly and in the work of Beverly Harrison, Rosemary Radford Reuther, Virginia Ramey Mollenkott, Phyllis Trible, Sallie McFague, Nancy Hardesty and others. Their claim that women have been historically excluded by language and practice is convincing. The time has come for women to be included. Inclusiveness, however, must not be regarded as only a feminist issue. Inclusiveness is a human concern. To act to be more inclusive of women is to act on behalf of men as well. We cannot be exclusive and whole at the same time.

Sallie McFague furthers the conversation:

> God as mother does not mean that God is mother (or father). We imagine God as both mother and father, but we realize how inadequate these and any other metaphors are to express the creative love of God, the love that gives, without calculating the return, the gift of the universe. Nevertheless, we speak of this love in language that is familiar and dear to us, the language of mothers and fathers who give us life, from whose bodies we come and upon whose care we depend. We in turn pass on that life, and in this model of birth, nurture, and fulfillment, we dimly perceive a pattern of giving and receiving in which to speak of God as creator.[5]

The Creator Is Both Transcendent and Imminent

To call God Creator is to observe the distinction between the one who creates and what is created. The created depends on the creator. The relationship between God and humanity is, therefore, dialogical rather than organic. It is the role of the creature to serve and worship the creator.

When this basic order is reversed, and humans worship the creature rather than the Creator, this is sin, and evil results (see Romans 1, esp. vv. 24-25). God's transcendence over creation, including humanity, means that our relationship is not contractual (an agreement among equals) but covenantal (an agreement among unequals), held together in an I-Thou relationship of benevolence on the part of the Creator and gratitude (Thanksgiving) on the part of the creature.

The transcendence of God marks the distinction of the Creator from the creature, and the immanence of God marks the presence of the Creator throughout creation without being identical with it. God is not identical with nature (pantheism) but present throughout its processes, from which God remains distinct.

It is important to observe both the transcendence and the immanence of God, and nowhere more so than in regard to healing. Healing stresses the immanence of God working through the processes of the person. Yet the person is ill at least in part precisely because her or his personal resources are inadequate to the demands of life. Transcendence offers the possibility of resources beyond those of the person that may come to his or her aid in healing. We shall speak more of this when we discuss grace and healing, but it is important to establish here that God is not only at work within the human psychophysical unit (including what Freud called the unconscious and what Jung called the collective unconscious) but also above and beyond it. God works through but is not reducible to the creation.

CREATION AS GIVEN AND AS GIFT

Creation may be regarded as a given or received as a gift. We may look upon nature as a given, as something that is simply "there." It is an object or a collection of objects. Indeed, the words *object* and *nature* are often linked, with *science* presented as an objective view of nature. This view extends to how we see ourselves within nature. We, too, are simply "there," part of nature with no clue to our origin or destiny. In the concept of one existentialist, we are thrown into the world like a marble in the mud. And the earth is there, thrown like a huge blue marble into the sky.

The Bible, however, proclaims that creation not only may be regarded as a given but also received as a gift. This is explicit in the Genesis stories where, after God has created the world and all that is in it, God turns it over to man and woman to care for the earth. They soon become careless, but then so do we.

Most of the time we take life for granted. We think life is a given. It's just here, that's all. It's not so much that we have it to live but that we have to live it. And one day seems very much like the day that's gone before it. Life is a given.

But then there are times when something happens, and the awful vulnerability of life is exposed. We see that every moment of our life is suspended over an abyss—an abyss of nothingness. We see then that it is only by a gift that each day comes to us, and in those moments we know that life is not a given. Life is a gift.

Life has been given to us, and life can be taken away from us. Illness is the crisis that brings home to us how fragile we are. We may be going along as if life were solid beneath our feet when cancer or a heart attack opens the trap door, and we find ourselves free-falling into an abyss of nothingness. If we are able to regain our footing, it never again seems quite so solid, for we know that every moment of our lives is suspended over this abyss. It is only as a gift that each day comes to us. When we come close to death, we know that life is not a given but a gift.

When was the moment you came closest to death? Recreating that experience of illness or accident is essential to remind us that our presence here is a gift of God's grace.

We exist by the very grace of God. Paul expresses this magnificently in Romans with these words: "For the wages of sin is death, but the free gift of God is eternal life in Christ Jesus our Lord" (Rom. 6:23). Life is a gift, and at any moment it may be taken from us. This is the truth about life, and all

that we give of ourselves is an offering back of what God has
given to us.

Life is much like breathing. When we inhale, we receive
the very air as a gift, and then we must exhale. The meaning
of life is to receive it as a gift and to offer it back as a gift. Out
of much anguish and searching I have come to this conclusion. How terrible it would be if we only breathed in, if we
were only receivers, if we were only takers. We would soon
become bloated and explode. Yes, we receive, but then we
give. We breathe out. We share the gift that has been given
to us.

This is so important that it is the basis of our life, the basis
of our stewardship. We are alive, thank God! Thank God!
That phrase comes to us spontaneously, for we sense in that
moment not only that life is a gift but also that God is the
giver.

Some may argue that this virtually universal experience is
not spontaneous but learned from those who already believe.
I do not agree. But even if this is a learned response, how is
it learned? It is learned out of just such experiences as this,
when life is threatened and offered back again.

God is surely proven not by thinking but by thanking.
Martin Heidegger believed that there is such a close relationship between thinking and thanking because our word *think*
derives from a word meaning "thanks." When we think
about God, we may "prove" God as an object of thought.
When we thank God, God is "proven" as a friend is "proven."
They are proven true. We can trust them.

This is not to disparage the proofs for the existence of God,
such as the cosmological and the ontological. These proofs
demonstrate a rational basis for belief in God. At the very
least they show that it is as rational to believe in God as not
to do so. But God as an object of thought cannot sustain us
on the journey of life. For this we seek a God who joins us on
the journey. The God of biblical faith is such a loving companion and not just a logical conclusion. When we sense that

we have such, we are tempted to cry out not "Eureka! I've found it," but "Thank God, God found me!" Life is a gift. There must be a giver, and God is that giver.

There is an admitted leap from "there must be a giver" to "God is the giver." This leap of faith was stressed by Sren Kierkegaard. He believed that the distinction between God and humanity was so deep that it could not be bridged but only leaped over. Nevertheless he spent a lot of time exploring just how the leap took place. This belief is an intuition, a direct perception into a transcendent order. Henri Bergson, the French philosopher, believed that this was as valid a basis for belief as scientific deduction.

I seriously doubt whether anyone who has never had the experience that "life is a gift, thank God!" can be argued into believing in God. But I also doubt whether anyone who has had this experience can be argued *out* of believing.

To believe that God is the giver of life is to believe that God stands apart from but in relation to us. The giver is not the gift. This is implicit in the biblical doctrine of creation. God is the Creator and, therefore, is not identical to the creation. Creation is a gift. Humanity is to care for this gift, and God speaks to the caretakers to guide them. The story of Noah and the flood dramatizes the way in which God creates a covenant with humanity to care for the earth. But something has gone wrong. The caretakers have become careless.

FREE TO CHOOSE

The essence of the Genesis story is that God has placed us in a cosmos rather than a chaos. There is order at the heart of life, which we can discover if we seek to do God's will. But disorder comes to our life when we disobey God. The story tells us that God creates the world to be good. The earth is there. The moon, the sun, the stars are there. The flora and the fauna are there. God sees all this and says, "It is good." It is "the way it is supposed to be." The boundaries are clearly set.

Then Adam and Eve come into the world. They are given the care of the earth, and they may wander freely throughout the garden, and they may eat of every tree except the tree of the knowledge of good and evil. That they must not touch. So, naturally, what do they do? Almost as soon as they can, Adam and Eve turn away from the whole garden in which they are free to move without any kind of penalty and head straight for the tree from which they have been forbidden to eat. Because they are disobedient, they learn, in fact, the knowledge of good and evil, and they are filled with shame; they become aware that they are naked. They had been naked before, but it was no bother; they were not aware of it. Out of their disobedience comes this awareness, which fractures life, creates disorder; everything goes awry.

We recognize ourselves in this story, or it would long ago have been forgotten. Are we not Adam and Eve? Have we not been given a life that is basically good and full of blessings? Have we not again and again by our own lust, greed, thirst for power, and hunger for control been disobedient and disordered life? Herein lies the root of our disease: We are broken from ourselves and from others because we are broken from God. Our souls are fractured long in advance of our bones.

Adam and Eve represent the propensity of human beings to want to enjoy all that God has given and do what is forbidden us. Bergson said that the earliest memory any of us has is the taste of forbidden fruit.

How did we acquire this taste? What is the source of our disease? One answer is Original Sin. This answer is capable of many interpretations, some sophisticated and others quite crude. But essentially it argues that human beings are disobedient by nature. Why do we do bad things? Because that's the way we are.

But Original Blessing is our birthright, others argue. At our core we are good. We may behave in ways disobedient and sinful, but at heart we are good, and we need only have this goodness brought out. This is the root of some contemporary approaches to healing.

To me, Original Freedom seems to be at the core of human nature. Human beings are neither good nor bad. They are their capacity to choose. On the basis of my reading of the biblical story and human experience, I agree with Jean-Paul Sartre that we are condemned to be free. Humans are their freedom. Choice is always ours. This is fundamental to human beings and, therefore, to the question of illness and healing. So radical is our freedom that even in the face of incapacitating illness we are free to choose how we will respond.

We are creatures; therefore, our life is conditioned. Our freedom is finite. We are not God, but we are made in the image of God. That is, we have the capacity to create. We create by the choices we make.

Our wellness rests on the use of our fragile freedom.

WELLNESS AND CREATION

The Genesis story addresses fundamental issues of health and healing from the perspective of faith in the God who creates. Wellness involves harmony with creation.

Wellness is an ingredient in God's creation. God's intention is for whole persons to live abundantly in a whole world. The person as a whole is symbolized by the blending of God's breath and the dust of the earth to form a biospiritual unity. The life abundant is symbolized in the companionship of male and female joining to become one flesh to care for each other and the earth. The whole world is symbolized by the cosmos that God creates out of chaos.

Health is a cosmic affair in that God creates with a purpose, and wellness is part of that purpose. God creates the world and places humans to live harmoniously in it and pronounces it "good"—the way it is supposed to be. There is a higher power in the universe, and aligning ourselves with that power contributes to our well-being, just as being out of alignment with that power contributes to our illness.

Health is cosmic also in that remedies for illness are to be found within nature as well as by manufacture or intervention. The latter approach is that of allopathic medicine, common in the West, in which treatment proceeds by finding something opposite to the condition. Homeopathic medicine, on the other hand, proceeds from feeling with the person and administering medication like that in the condition in judicious amounts. These two approaches have been opposed for many years. (At the present time, some homeopathic elements are being incorporated into mainstream allopathic practice, for example, the use of medicinal herbs.)

Healing as a cosmic activity is foreign to allopathic medicine, but at home in alternative approaches throughout the world, such as in Asian and Native American medicine. Such alternative approaches around the world rest on the concept of the planet as a living organism. According to Stanley Krippner and Patrick Welch, although allopathic and homeopathic medicines are very different and historically opposed, they are not necessarily incompatible. They conclude their book *Spiritual Dimensions of Healing* with chapters on integrating spiritual healing into counseling and psychotherapy and into nursing and medicine. Bill Moyers's television program "Healing and the Mind" visualizes much of this process from another perspective.

Theodore Roszak has redefined the very meaning of health within an environmental context. In *The Voice of the Earth,* Roszak shows that personal neurosis can be traced to the abuse of the planetary environment by drawing on the works of psychologists, ecologists, theologians, and modern cosmologists. If we are to be healed, therefore, we must heal our relationship to the earth.

Thus, as foreign as it may seem at first, the Genesis view of health and healing as cosmic activities is becoming a key to the new medicine. The earth-care issue is a health-care issue.

TO CARE FOR OUR HEALTH, WE MUST CARE FOR THE EARTH

Ideally, humans would care for the earth simply because they believe in Father God or Mother Earth. That ideal is shattered by the appalling devastation of the planet, evident in the pollution of the water and the air, destruction of rain forests, acid rain, and other disasters. The reality now is that we must end our exploitation of the earth or the exploitation will end us.

Norman Cousins did much to draw public attention to social issues. Over the years Cousins has written a dozen books on the ills of nations, and all of them combined have not received the response of his account of his personal bout with illness in *Anatomy of an Illness.* The irony was not lost on Cousins, who did not complain about it or deny the importance of individual health. He wrote, "What concerns me is that everyone's health—including that of the next generation—may depend more on the health of society and the healing of nations than on the conquest of disease."[6]

In *The Healing Heart,* Cousins identified a series of health hazards that were brought on by society itself, including the manufacture and sale of handguns and other killing devices, society's attitude toward automobile and highway safety, the manufacture and sale of lethal sprays and insecticides, and, at the top of the ladder, the combustible way in which nations conduct their affairs with one another. He concludes the book, which begins with the story of his massive heart attack, with these words: "The health and well-being not just of Americans but of the human race are incompatible with war and preparation for war. The conquest of war, therefore, must become our grand preoccupation and magnificent obsession."[7]

In the Genesis story, God created humans in the divine image to care for the earth and have dominion over living things (Gen. 1:26). The agenda, then, was to till and keep the garden, to be fruitful, and to fill and subdue the earth. The human agenda must still be to care for the earth, although being fruitful and multiplying and subduing the earth are no longer consistent with caring for the earth; in fact, they are counterproductive to it. A new agenda to this end is set forth by Al Gore in his book *Earth in the Balance*. This work is essential for understanding what we must do in our time to care for the earth and why we must do it. In the conclusion, Gore tells why he has written the book and where we may start in enacting the program he sets forth:

> If it is possible to steer one's own course—and I do believe it is—then I am convinced that the place to start is with faith, which for me is akin to a kind of spiritual gyroscope that spins in its own circumference in a stabilizing harmony with what is inside and what is out. Of course, faith is just a word unless it is invested with personal meaning; my own faith is rooted in the unshakeable belief in God as creator and sustainer, a deeply personal interpretation of and relationship with Christ, and an awareness of a constant and holy spiritual presence in all people, all life, and all things. But I also want to affirm what people of faith from long ago apparently knew and that our civilization has obscured: that there is revelatory power in the world. This is the essence of faith: to make a surrendering decision to invest belief in a spiritual reality larger than ourselves. And I believe that faith is the primary force that enables us to choose meaning and direction and then hold to it despite all the buffeting chaos in life.[8]

This passage on how faith in the God who creates, redeems, and sustains us and leads us from chaos to cosmos not only is a fitting conclusion to this chapter but also an expression of our main theme.

CHAPTER
F I V E

GOD'S LOVE REDEEMS:
Jesus Christ on "Larry King Live"

Larry King is one of the most influential men today as the host of television and radio interview shows with audiences around the world. Powerful people stand in line to appear on his shows, but King has said that if he could invite anyone from all of history to appear on his television show he would turn not to the rich and famous but to Jesus Christ. "I would ask him if he believed that he was born of virgin birth, because whatever the answer is changes or reinforces the world," King said.

That Larry King would choose Jesus Christ as his most desired interview guest is a measure of Christ's fascination, and that King would ask him a theological question is a measure of Christ's mystery. Fundamental to this fascination and mystery is the redeeming work of Jesus Christ. Jesus was a great historical figure. Yet if he were only that, he might be enshrined in a tomb like Lenin. Instead, for nearly two thousand years men and women have worshiped him as a living Lord and Savior.

Who is this Jesus Christ, and what has he to do with healing today?

That Jesus Christ is regarded as the Great Physician is fundamental to his enduring appeal. Jesus' healing power is not something added to his being but the natural expression

73

and overflow of his life. Jesus' vitality is so enormous that even now people speak of him in the present tense, as I will.

Few people have seen the connection between Jesus' life force and his healing more clearly than Wilhelm Reich, M.D., an early student and colleague of Freud and teacher of Alexander Lowen. Reich's *The Murder of Christ* is a neglected classic. Jesus radiated energy (Reich called it orgone energy) so powerfully that it excited the "dead" energy systems of those in misery. Reich wrote:

> This induced excitation of the weak living system is experienced as relief from tenseness and anxiety, due to the expansion of the nervous system, and it even provides a quiet, kindly, lovely glow of true love in an otherwise hateful organism. The excited bioenergy in the weak is capable of expanding the blood vessels, of including better blood supply to the tissues, of improving the healing of wounds, of counteracting the stale, degenerative effects of stagnant life energy.[1]

According to Reich, people filled themselves up with the strength and "radiating loveliness of Christ, like men dying of thirst seep up water from a well," and this was the secret of Jesus' healing power. This healing power is still available today through the church, which is truly the body of Christ, and through Christ's mystical presence at large in the world, often incognito.

Jesus' passion for life survives even the passion of his death. He lives, he loves, he works, he studies, he cares, and he gives himself to his belief without reservation. He embraces life with its joys and sorrows and lifts it all into the light of the divine. In Jesus Christ, God meets us in our highest hopes and in our deepest needs and shows us how to celebrate life.

It is true that not everyone has found this belief compelling, and that crimes have been committed by some who have claimed to be followers of Christ. Jesus has appeared as less appealing than this description. Nietzsche, for one, found him a weakling. But I agree with James Agee, who, commenting on a film version of Jesus Christ's life, said that Christ did not creep. In the passion with which he lived and the dignity with which he died, many people in every age and every land have seen in Jesus Christ what human beings are meant to be.

JESUS CHRIST: OUR REDEEMER

If Jesus Christ is such a powerful figure on purely human terms, why would Larry King want to ask about his birth from a virgin? Because for nearly two thousand years people who have come into contact with Jesus have been aware that purely human terms cannot account for the presence of the divine in Jesus, and the virgin birth has been a primary symbol of this presence. Actually, this doctrine is only one way of trying to express the conviction that Jesus Christ is God with us. In Jesus Christ we are dealing with ultimate reality. We are dealing with God, not a being like God, but "very God of very God" as well as "very man of very man," as one creed puts it.

How Jesus Christ is at once fully human and fully divine is a mystery that no doctrine can explain. Americans often like to think of the typical success story in which a person goes from rags to riches. In Jesus Christ we find just the reverse. Here, God exchanged the richness of divine sovereignty for the rags of human suffering. Why? Second Corinthians 8:9 puts it succinctly: "Though he was rich, yet for your sakes he became poor, so that by his poverty you might become rich."

I once went to call in a home burdened with suffering. At the door I was met by the mother of a young woman who was then in the hospital undergoing delicate surgery and lay near death. Feeling deeply the limits of words at such a time, I quietly commented, "All we can do now is pray." The mother replied with wet eyes, "Oh, I have been praying. I've been praying all the time. At night I pull up a chair by the side of my bed and invite God to sit there as I talk with him."

In Jesus Christ, God pulls up a chair by the bedside of suffering and whispers, "There is hope." There is hope because there is One with us who is yet more than we, and by his suffering we are healed.

God is present with us in our joys and sorrows. However abstract it may sound, to refer to Christ as the second person of the Trinity is to say that the love of Christ is none other than the love of God, who creates and sustains as well as redeems us. In his book *The Christian Understanding of God*, Nels F. S. Ferré says that Jesus Christ shows conclusively God's "nature of love both as being and becoming." He adds:

> What matters is that God himself operates healingly in history, forgiving our sins and offering us newness of life in terms of which wrongs are restored and a new level of fellowship attained. . . . This enactment of the love of God is through and through by his very nature atoning, vicarious, redemptive.[2]

The enduring fascination of Jesus Christ rests in his being the pattern and the power by which we are to live. Jesus Christ is not only our role model but also our redeemer.

To say that God's love redeems is to acknowledge that humans stand in need of redemption. The purpose intended by God's good creation has been thwarted. By our own action, we humans are separated from the source of our being and, therefore, from ourselves and others. A word from the city streets captures what humans have done. Among street gangs, the ultimate insult is to show disrespect for another, and if one is "dissed," death may be the price one pays for the act. Humans have "dissed" God; we have defined our relationship in the negative. We have shown disrespect, disobedience, and the result is disorientation and disease. We are lost, and we are sick. How are we to find our way home and be healed?

The human predicament is such that the more we struggle to find our way, the more lost we become. Our condition is like that of the men whose plane went down in the wilds of New Guinea where they were completely lost. Fortunately, a native man who knew some English appeared. "Show us the way," they cried. The man answered, "I am the way." Then he led them through the uncharted wilderness to safety.

There are situations in which our lostness is so extreme that only the personal presence of a guide can lead us out. That is the human condition as perceived by faith. Humanity has wandered so far from its source that there is no way back. There is only the One who comes from the source itself and declares, "I am the Way," who can lead us home. Jesus Christ made that claim to his disciples. Then, and in every generation since, persons have made their way to home and health under that guidance.

At the heart of the Christian faith, there is a person—not a plan, a program, an institution, or a doctrine—a person named Jesus Christ.

THE HEART OF CHRISTIANITY

The life and teaching of Jesus have been the subject of many books. Is it possible to sum them up succinctly? Whether or not there is an essence of Christianity has occupied countless scholars, who have come up with no universally accepted answer. The question is admittedly difficult. Yet, Jesus himself was asked the question, and he answered it.

A lawyer asked Jesus, "Which commandment in the law is the greatest?" Jesus replied, " 'You shall love the Lord your God with all your heart, and with all your soul, and with all your mind.' This is the greatest and first commandment. And a second is like it: 'You shall love your neighbor as yourself.'

On these two commandments hang all the law and the prophets" (Matt. 22:36-40).

Jesus reveals that the heart of Christianity is the Christianity of the heart. Love is the core from which everything flows and to which it returns.

Jesus identifies three dimensions that are distinct yet interrelated: Love of God, love of neighbor, and love of self. The distinctions are important because without all three love is incomplete. The interrelationship is important because the quality of one affects the others. Kierkegaard saw this when he wrote:

> If anyone, therefore, will not learn from Christianity to love himself in the right way, then neither can he love his neighbor. . . . To love oneself in the right way and to love one's neighbor are absolutely analogous concepts, are at bottom one and the same. . . . Hence the law is: "You shall love yourself as you love your neighbor when you love him as yourself."[3]

These three loves are not sequential but simultaneous. One does not first love God, then one's neighbor, followed by oneself; rather, in the act of truly loving God, one loves one's neighbor and oneself.

The question may be asked, "But how can we love if it is commanded by God?" Carl Michalson answered this with another question: "How can we love if it were not commanded by God?" This teacher was claiming that love is not a sentiment we may or may not feel but a commandment. We love not because we feel like it but because God asks it of us, and the God who asks us to love is the God who loves us. Our love is grounded in the divine love, enabling us to love even what is not lovely.

This is why it is so important that Jesus not only taught love but also lived love. God's act of love in Christ empowers us to love. God's love initiates our love. As John put it, "We love because he first loved us." The heart of Christianity is the Christianity of the heart.

JESUS CHRIST LIVED AND TAUGHT LOVE

Jesus never defined love in his teaching. This makes answering the question "What is the heart of Christianity?" so problematical. The question almost invariably seeks a different kind of answer. A precise, clear definition—Jesus simply never gave one; nor did Paul, who declared that love is the greatest thing in the world; nor did John, who said that God is love.

This lack of definition for the word is intentional. Offer a definition, and the intellect takes over and starts analyzing the word. By not offering a formal definition of *love*, Jesus presents love as something to be lived rather than analyzed. In his life, Jesus defined love. If one wants to find the meaning of love, consider the life of Jesus.

Jesus lives love. He takes the noisy children into his arms and says, "Of such is the kingdom of heaven." He comes upon the woman taken in adultery and declares, "Let him who is without sin cast the first stone." He reaches out to the outcasts, the sick, the lepers and invites them into the Kingdom of God. He reaches out to all of life and embraces it. This love will prove too threatening for the lives of many human beings and will lead him at last to the cross. But even there he will cry out, "Father, forgive them." And at last his love will prove stronger than death. "Herein is love, not that we loved God but that God loved us." This is the heart of Christianity, the core from which everything flows.

When we try to trace the circulation of love, we discover that love lives by loving—that is, love reveals itself in acts of love.

We also discover that the love that is in Jesus Christ is relational not only to us but also to God as Creator and Holy Spirit. The love of Jesus is understood from the beginning not as an isolated fragment but as a revelation of the very heart of God. "See what love the Father has given us, that we should be called children of God" (1 John 3:1).

And love finds its fulfillment through the Spirit. Formal doctrines of the Trinity come later, but they have their root in the love of God and the faces or personae of love God presents to us.

THE LIMITS OF LOVE

There is much talk today about unconditional love. But truly unconditional love is possible only for God, because only God is unconditioned. All human love is conditioned to some extent. God is the unconditioned ground of all conditioned human love. Recognizing the limits of human love enriches rather than impoverishes it. When unconditional love is made a prerequisite for healing, it may have the opposite effect because we fall short. Unconditional love may mean that the lover does not love on condition that his or her love be returned, or that the lover loves another no matter what his or her condition may be. In these and other cases, unconditional love is a useful term. But when loving without limits is made the norm for human behavior, it becomes self-defeating. We rarely, if ever, find such love, let alone create it, and the effort can make us sick.

The unconditioned love we long for, the love that loves us without limits, is available but can be found only in God. To be made perfect in this love is our aim, but as John Wesley said, in this life we are "going on to perfection." Love that acts on behalf of the beloved within the limits of the lover and of the beloved is no less real for being limited. Furthermore, valuing conditioned love frees us from demanding or even expecting unconditional love from others. On what basis did we expect unconditional love from our parents anyway? We can accept the love of our parents and others, however imperfect it may be, because we know that they have been conditioned by their parents and other circumstances in their lives. To paraphrase John Wesley, we can share all the love we can with all the people we can as long as we can and rejoice as often as we can for receiving the love that comes our way, however imperfect it may be.

There are limits to love. Nevertheless, within the limits, love is still the greatest value, the most worthy goal, and the preferred way of living for faith. Love gives us a passion for life at its highest and compassion when we fall short.

This is the meaning of life for me: to try to honor such love and to love in spite of all the unloveliness in and around me. This is the love I see in Jesus Christ.

If we ask, "How could a person so full of life and love be condemned to death on the cross?" we might well answer, "For that very reason." The radiant energy of Jesus Christ eventually proved too threatening to the brittle religious and political institutions of his day, so they tried to extinguish it by putting him to death. For whatever reason, Jesus was crucified. But so powerful was he that he took the ugliest form of death known to the ancient world—death by the torture of crucifixion—and transformed it into a symbol of life and beauty.

In Jesus' body, broken on the cross, humanity finds healing for its brokenness.

THE WAY OF THE CROSS

The cross stands for the act whereby God at great cost gave his Son to bring rebellious humans back to the divine purpose. This reconciling act of God is called atonement. The meaning of this word is made clear simply by pronouncing it slowly: *at-one-ment*. The meaning of the cross is that here God takes love to the limits so that humans may be at one with God, with others, and with themselves.

It is obvious that we are not at one; we live broken lives in the midst of a broken world. If sickness is a dysfunction between the parts of a system, then we live in a sick world. Healing, therefore, must be not only a correction of personal dysfunction but also a connection with holistic function. To say that God's love redeems us is to say that God has acted to restore order to the universe and empower us to recover from our disobedience and disease.

The source of our personal and social chaos lies in our brokenness from God. Although we do not often think in such terms, many of us are aware that we are cut off from the center of life itself. There is great power in the world, but we are not powerful. There is great love in the world, but we are not loving. There is great beauty in the world, but we are not beautiful. We are not at one with the primal, spontaneous joy at the heart of things. We are not at one with God.

We are obviously not at one with one another. The brokenness of our relationships is brought home to us not only by the report of gun shots from abroad or on our streets but also by the clink of a coffee cup against the saucer on our table when we look at someone we love and sense an awful gulf between ourselves and them.

Regrettably, we are not at one with ourselves. We may feel a frightful range of possibilities in our lives but be unable to find our real self among them. Or we may feel that the possibilities we have are so limited that we crack. Many people are like the elevator girl in the motion picture *The Apartment* who carried a broken mirror in her purse. "It makes me look the way I feel," she explained.

These are signs of our brokenness, but the cross means that God has not left us here alone. Saint Augustine said that the cross is a plank that God has flung across the sea of the world to connect with us. The cross means that we may be at one with God, with other people, and with ourselves.

The cross means that God loves us. John 3:16 tells us, "For God so loved the world, that he gave his only begotten Son, that whosoever believeth in him should not perish, but have everlasting life" (KJV). One of the first Christians to fully grasp this meaning of the cross was Irenaeus, the Bishop of Lyon, who lived in the second century. Irenaeus looked on the cross and said, "Behold, how he loved us." God's act in Christ has been the free, uninhibited outpouring of his inmost nature. "The Son has revealed the Father in his love."

We need this love of God. A woman said to me the most pathetic words I think I've ever heard: "Nobody cares whether I live or die." Most of us feel this way at one time or another. We need to know that someone cares about us. God cares. Our lives matter to God. How do we know this? We read it on the cross. The cross is God's love letter to the world, written on wood, engraved by nails, signed in blood, saying, "God loves you." God loves us because it is his "nature" to love. He will keep on loving us until everything that stands between him and us is consumed by the intensity of his passion.

If the love of God were merely a single and isolated act, we might try to get rid of it, like a young woman burning the love letters of a former suitor. But because the love of God is as eternally present as God, it exerts a constant pressure on our lives to be at one with God.

The divine love is like human love in that it must be simply accepted to be shared. It is unlike human love in that it never fails. In the spring, young girls pick flowers and anxiously tear off the petals, whispering, "He loves me, he loves me not. . . ." There is no such uncertainty with God. We may look at the strangest flower God ever planted, the cross, and say with utter certainty, "God loves me."

The cross means that God lifts us. Jesus said, "I, if I be lifted up, will draw all people unto me." Anselm, one of the great Christian thinkers of the twelfth century, found that the cross means that God has done for us what we could never do for ourselves.

Anselm looked on the cross and perceived that human sinfulness is so profound that even our best acts are defective. Our brokenness from God is so complete that our efforts to redeem ourselves only cause us to sink more deeply into the quicksand of our own treachery. Only God can save us by entering the quicksand to offer us a secure foothold, a way out, and a new status in life. God lifts us.

Nevertheless, we humans try frantically to lift ourselves. There are at least two ways in which we may be lifted. Some people try to lift themselves up by the way of force. They try to elevate themselves by their own ambition. They try to lift themselves by their own self-will and moral effort. But they rise to fall again.

Then there is the way of the cross. The cross lifts us. We look at the cross and the Son of God upon it, and it draws us toward him with an undeniable authority. We are lifted above the soiled streams of self-concern into the deep, strong currents of eternal love. Christ reaches out from the cross to lift us from our littleness and to place our feet on the high places of the will of God.

The elevating power of the descending God makes its force known in our personal relationship with God, but it also lifts our fellow humans. "I, if I be lifted up, will draw *all people* unto me." The God who does for us what we cannot do for ourselves helps us to do for ourselves what we cannot do without God. God has entered human life not only to free us from our sin, but also to offer us a foothold in the midst of our sin. What we can never do merely in our own power—namely, love one another—we are empowered to do through the love of God, which comes to us in Christ. The grace of God is as essential to the salvation of society as it is to the salvation of individuals. God descends into human life to lift *all people.* And if all are not lifted by God's gracious act, no one will be lifted.

The cross means that God leads us. Jesus said, "Whoever does not carry the cross and follow me cannot be my disciple" (Luke 14:27). Peter Abelard, a great Christian thinker of the twelfth century, gave the idea of Christ the Pattern its classic expression.

Looking on the cross, Abelard perceived in Christ the vision of perfect humanity as well as perfect divinity. The love of Christ awakens in the human a sense of dissatisfaction with self and moves one to become like Christ. Martin Luther later put this wisely when he said, "It is not by imitating that we become sons. But by becoming sons we become also imitators." No one can really see Christ without longing to be like him.

We need the kind of discipleship that gives a compelling vision to our lives. We need to follow Christ. We wander aimlessly until we do. We need that of which we can say, "For this I was born. To this I can give my life, my all, everything." We can say this of the way of the cross. As Christ's disciples, his purpose becomes our purpose, his will becomes our will. At last the one consuming purpose of our lives is to live as he lived and to love as he loved.

If we are not at one with ourselves, we have not found the way of the cross. The brokenness of our lives can be healed not by pulling ourselves together but by being pulled together by a compelling power. What we need is not a kind of psychic cement that tentatively brings together the disparate elements of our broken personalities, but a magnetic force that draws us into dynamic wholeness. The life of Christ is such a magnetic force, and the way of the cross, just because it is narrow, is the way to integration of the self.

The "image of the self" is a phrase much used these days, with good reason. Everyone has an image of self around which one consciously and unconsciously attempts to organize one's life. We suffer because most of us cannot accept the self-image conferred on us by our parents, and we cannot discover in our commercialized culture a vision of ourselves that has unifying power. If our self-image is broken, our daily lives can do no more than reflect this brokenness.

The place to seek our true self-image is not in the broken mirrors of our culture, but in the face of Jesus Christ, who is not only God in divine perfection but also human in his potentiality. Christ can offer the human being the self-image that can unify one's life. There is no way but the way of the cross in which one can be at one with oneself.

The way of the cross is at first the way of self-surrender. It means the abandonment of our fond, foolish hopes for fulfillment. The most profound words ever spoken about human personality were uttered by Jesus: "Those who want to save their life will lose it, and those who lose their life for my sake will find it" (Matt. 16:25).

We lay a broken self at the foot of the cross. We rise a whole person to take up our cross. On the pilgrimage to wholeness, God leads us. Being one with God makes being one with ourselves and others possible.

The resurrection of Jesus Christ means that this wholeness embraces death itself, as we shall see in the next chapter. Now let us attend to how the forgiveness granted by God may become real in healing.

FORGIVENESS AND HEALING

The healing power of Jesus Christ comes to a crux where guilt meets grace. Said Nels Ferré: "The world today is suffering from unforgiven guilt. In vain we wash our hands in the milk of human kindness." Unforgiven guilt is one of the greatest problems in the world, destroying nations that nurse ancient hatreds as surely as individuals who cannot forgive themselves. I am speaking now of inappropriate or neurotic guilt. Every individual and community needs boundaries of acceptable behavior, and when those boundaries are crossed, guilt and punishment are appropriate.

Inappropriate guilt makes people sick. This may be true for specific ailments, as when feelings of guilt lead to gastric ulcers or other physical disturbances. But this is also true in a more basic way when one feels unworthy to be fully healthy and alive. Such persons may punish themselves unmercifully and undercut the very possibility of good health.

Jesus Christ had a profound sense of the connection between guilt and illness. He made forgiveness the key to his ministry of healing. Almost invariably when someone presented a physical complaint to him, Jesus responded with the words, "Your sins are forgiven."

Healing and forgiveness are deeply related. This is shown dramatically in the case of a paralyzed man who was brought to Jesus by his friends. They could not get in through the door of the house where Jesus was, so they went up on the roof and lowered the man on his bed into Jesus' presence. Jesus' first comment was, "Friend, your sins are forgiven."

That seems like a strange approach. The scribes and Pharisees who were there found it strange because they believed that only God could forgive sins, and therefore Jesus was speaking blasphemy. We may find it strange that forgiveness was linked with healing at all. What has one to do with the other?

To begin to understand the answer to this question, we must determine what we mean by *sin*. If we mean acts we ought not perform, then the association with healing would be arbitrary. But if by sins we mean whatever separates us from God, then forgiveness is necessary.

Sin may express itself in the flesh or social injustice or greed or crime or some other obvious act. But sin is primarily that attitude of the prideful ego that seeks to put itself in the place of Almighty God, and by doing so distances itself from God.

Sin, then, is actions that express our separation from God and wall us off from the divine. When we are forgiven, those blocks are removed and the divine energy is able to flow once again, opening up the possibility of being healed, being whole. Once the relationship between the divine and the human is restored, the power to heal is released. This is why forgiveness is essential to healing.

Complex though the process of forgiveness is, there is a central issue. To the one who asks, "How may I be forgiven?"

the answer is "As you forgive others." This is drawn from the Lord's prayer. Jesus taught us to pray, "Forgive us our trespasses as we forgive those who trespass against us." Our forgiveness of others is a different process from the forgiveness of our own trespasses, but these processes are so closely related that to experience the one is to know the other. When we are able to forgive fully those who have hurt us, we feel ourselves fully forgiven.

When we have faith that God loves us so much that God has broken down the wall between us, we no longer maintain the walls between ourselves and others. In the act of forgiving others, we know ourselves to be forgiven by the God to whom we have prayed for forgiveness.

Forgiveness does not mean condoning behavior, either your own or that of another. Forgiveness means accepting God's love and letting go of your hurt, making restitution when possible with whomever you blamed for it or whomever you hurt, and moving on with your life.

Forgiveness means accepting responsibility for what you did and who you are and putting an end to blame. Forgiveness means living by the words, "If we confess our sins, [God] who is faithful and just will forgive us our sins and cleanse us from all unrighteousness" (1 John 1:9). "If we walk in the light as he himself is in the light, we have fellowship with one another, and the blood of Jesus his Son cleanses us from all sin" (1 John 1:7).

Nothing greater than being forgiven can happen to a human being, according to Paul Tillich. He writes in *The New Being*: "Forgiveness means reconciliation in spite of estrangement; it means reunion in spite of hostility; it means acceptance of those who are unacceptable, and it means reception of those who are rejected." This is made possible because of God's forgiveness of our sins through Jesus Christ. Tillich writes that when we accept our acceptance by God even though we are unacceptable, then "like a fiery stream, His healing power enters into us; we can affirm Him and with

Him our own being and the others from whom we were estranged and live as a whole.

"Forgiveness is the answer, the divine answer, to the question implied in our existence," Tillich continues.[4] However, once forgiveness is accepted as the answer to the question of our existence, the question remains as to how that forgiveness becomes existential for us. The church acknowledges this in sacraments and rituals with acts of confession and repentance.

For many people, guilt lies so deep and forgiveness comes with such difficulty that therapy is needed. The fact that guilt contributes to sickness and forgiveness contributes to wellness is agreed upon by virtually all the professionals in the field. So overwhelming is this consensus that documenting it would constitute a huge volume. Here I will simply identify some major resources and urge you to pursue them:

- "Guilt is the Wound, Love is the Healer" is the way Joan Borysenko expresses it in her book *Guilt Is the Teacher, Love Is the Lesson* (New York: Warner Books, 1990). She has developed a way of "minding the body, mending the mind" based on this insight, which she describes in her book by the same title (New York: Bantam, 1988).

- Dr. Jerry Jampolski addresses guilt through his "attitudinal healing," which connects the themes of his books *Teach Only Love: The Seven Principles of Attitudinal Healing* (Toronto: Bantam, 1983) and *Goodbye to Guilt* (Toronto: Bantam, 1985). Dr. Jampolski has done important work on love and healing, especially with young cancer patients. See his book *Out of Darkness, into the Light: A Journey of Inner Healing* (New York: Bantam, 1989).

- Shame also cripples. Whereas guilt tends to find root in specific "wrongs" we have done, shame is a toxic reaction to who we are. John Bradshaw creatively confronts this shame, which is a root cause of addiction and codependency, in *Healing the Shame That Binds You* (Deerfield Beach, Fla.: Health Communications, 1988), a guidebook for breaking free.

One thing is clear, whether guilt and/or shame underlie our illness and whatever the mode of therapy, we are not likely to hear the words "Stand up and walk" until we have heard "Your sins are forgiven."

As I was working on the manuscript for this book, I found myself badly blocked on the subject of guilt and forgiveness. I was trying to write about grace, but I did not feel much of it. Why did I feel so much more guilt than grace?

The immediate issue was guilt. I did not believe that I deserved to feel grace because I was behind on my writing schedule. But I also felt that I had fallen behind in other areas of my life as well. I found myself thinking in some twisted fashion like this: "I don't deserve God's grace, so I will punish myself until I am caught up with my work, and then I will allow myself to feel God's grace!"

At that point an image came to me of the tunnel that connects the parking lot and my favorite ocean beach. The beach is beautiful, but the tunnel stinks, literally. It is dark, water often leaks in from above, and animal waste is not uncommon below. Yet here I was acting as if I had a day at the beach and were spending it in the tunnel. I was allowing myself to get stuck in the tunnel of guilt.

This symbolized my situation—not only in that moment but at other times in my life, and not only for myself but for many people I know as well. With the light of a beautiful beach shining not far away, we condemn ourselves to imprisonment in the dark, stinking tunnel. How are we to get out? It is not as simple as it sounds. If it were, we would be out. Instead, there is some fascination with the dark that holds us, and the desire to be out does not deliver us.

We get out because Someone comes to us in the tunnel of our despair to show us that we are loved just as we are and just where we are, however dark and stinking that may be. We are loved just as we are, the work not done, the house not in order, the tasks not finished. You are loved just as you are, here and now. You are free to come out of the darkness into the light. If you want to walk out and play on the beach, you are free to do so now. Come, walk in the light! If you wish to stay here, you may. It is up to you.

When I do leave the tunnel imaginatively, when I let go, when I leave my baggage behind and walk into the light, immediately grace is everywhere. Grace is in the air. It is all around me: in the sky, the trees, the birds, the breeze, my food, my friends, my work, my play. I do not have to earn this grace. In fact, I cannot earn it. But I do not need to postpone it. I do not need to punish myself. I can let the light shine in now, in the midst of the unfinished business, when I most need it.

Since that revelation, I feel different. I know that I can postpone the experience of grace if I choose. I may stay in my darkness and guilt. But I know that Someone has come to me in the darkness and to show me the way out, and I am free to walk out and live in that light whenever I choose.

Grace is greater than guilt when I let go of fear and give way to love.

Who is Jesus Christ, and what has he to do with healing today? Jesus Christ was a historical figure who is experienced by believers as a contemporary presence, the bearer of God's eternal love. Jesus Christ lives and teaches love, divine and human. Healing expressions of this love are found in Jesus Christ's power to forgive sins and elicit faith, awaken the self, strengthen the will to live, and encourage creativity in the face of suffering. In all this, Jesus Christ is the Redeemer, leading us to our eternal source, bringing atonement with the Creator, and showing us the way to be whole again.

CHAPTER
SIX

GOD'S LOVE SUSTAINS:
The Holy Spirit and the Healthy Body

The Holy Spirit was referred to by Jesus as the Comforter. To test how powerful this comfort may be, let us explore in this chapter its ramifications, including confrontation with illness and death.

It is the work of the Holy Spirit to make present the healing power of Christ and of the Creator without drawing attention to itself. In Hebrew and Aramaic, which was Jesus' native tongue, the word used for "spirit" is *ruach*, which means "breath" or "wind."

Jesus associated the wind and the Spirit in his conversation with Nicodemus, as recorded in the Gospel of John. Nicodemus was a ruler of the Jews, a celebrity so well known that he came to Jesus by night to avoid publicity. Nicodemus had everything—and he had nothing. He had succeeded in the flesh but failed spiritually, and he came to Jesus hoping, no doubt, that he could quickly obtain some of the miraculous power that Jesus had exhibited.

Jesus set him straight when he said, "You must be born anew." Jesus told Nicodemus that what he needed was blowing in the wind. The wind is free, and although it cannot be seen it can be experienced. It blows wherever it wills. We hear its sound, but we cannot tell where it comes from or where it is going. People who are born of the Spirit are like that.

There is no direct account of Nicodemus's immediate response. But he showed up at the cross and was helpful in the aftermath. He must have come to believe that when Jesus said, "God so loved the world, that he gave his only begotten Son, that whosoever believeth in him should not perish, but have everlasting life" (John 3:16 KJV), Jesus was talking about him.

What Jesus said to Nicodemus, Christ says to us today: "You must be born anew." We must take the passage from the material realm to the spiritual, and that is as traumatic as birth itself.

Yet this passage is essential if we are to be made whole. The person who wants to be healed must die to one way of life and be born to another. This way of life renews the old by embodying a new spirit.

THE HOLY SPIRIT, JESUS, AND HEALING

The Holy Spirit is associated with Jesus and healing so constantly that these themes are virtually inseparable.

They are sufficiently separable to establish the Holy Spirit as distinct from the Son, but theologians have been careful not to make that separation too great. The doctrines of Jesus' conception by the Holy Spirit and birth of the Virgin Mary may be regarded as a way of symbolizing the direct and immediate relationship among Father, Son, and Holy Spirit.

Doctrinal matters such as this did not become explicit until the fourth century when the church was trying systematically to clarify its understanding of the signs and wonders of God's action. These signs and wonders themselves are the main subject matter of the New Testament.

At the very beginning of Jesus' public ministry, the continuity and discontinuity with Judaism, the presence of the Spirit, and healing come together. Luke reports it:

Then Jesus, filled with the power of the Spirit, returned to Galilee, and a report about him spread through all the surrounding country. He began to teach in their synagogues and was praised by everyone. When he came to Nazareth, where he had been brought up, he went to the synagogue on the sabbath day, as was his custom. He stood up to read, and the scroll of the prophet Isaiah was given to him. He unrolled the scroll and found the place where it was written:
> "The Spirit of the Lord is upon me,
> because he has anointed me
> to bring good news to the poor.
> He has sent me to proclaim release
> to the captives
> and recovery of sight to the blind,
> to let the oppressed go free,
> to proclaim the year of the Lord's favor."

And he rolled up the scroll, gave it back to the attendant, and sat down. The eyes of all in the synagogue were fixed on him. Then he began to say to them, "Today this scripture has been fulfilled in your hearing." (Luke 4:14-21)

This pattern of events recurs throughout Jesus' ministry, and at the end Jesus again speaks explicitly about the Holy Spirit as a continuing presence in ministry. John reports a "farewell speech" in which Jesus faces his own death and seeks to console his troubled disciples. Jesus says, "I will ask the Father, and he will give you another Advocate, to be with you forever. This is the Spirit of truth" (John 14:16-17a).

The Holy Spirit descended upon the disciples "with a sound like the rush of a violent wind" on the Day of Pentecost (Acts 2:2). There was a great outpouring of the Holy Spirit with ecstatic experiences, and out of this event the church was forged as a community committed to carrying on the ministry of Jesus. That communal life has four major marks or activities: studying the apostles' teaching (*didache*), fellowship (*koinonia*), breaking of bread (*diakonia*), and worship (*leitourgia*).

Preaching and healing are at the center of Christian life and witness. Peter's preaching defines the event of Pentecost, and the first activity recorded in Acts once the community is formed is that of Peter and John healing a lame man by the Beautiful Gate in a way that echoes Jesus' healing of the man by the pool of Bethesda.

Healing was carried on within the Christian community as well. James sets forth a prescription for healing that must have been a description of familiar, even ritual, occurrences:

> Are any among you suffering? They should pray. Are any cheerful? They should sing songs of praise. Are any among you sick? They should call for the elders of the church and have them pray over them, anointing them with oil in the name of the Lord. The prayer of faith will save the sick, and the Lord will raise them up. . . . Therefore confess your sins to one another, and pray for one another, so that you may be healed. The prayer of the righteous is powerful and effective. (James 5:13-16)

This mission of preaching and healing carried through the apostolic age, according to one of its leading scholars, G. B. Caird. He writes in *The Apostolic Age:*

> For the Epistles bear their concurrent witness that the preaching of the Gospel was everywhere accompanied by exorcisms and healings and by other forms of miracle which are expressly distinguished from miraculous cures. . . . At that time their mission had been an extension of Jesus' own ministry of preaching and healing. The healing work of the early church was a continuation of the same ministry, carried on in the name of Jesus and in the power of his presence. Particularly significant are the words of Peter to Aeneas: "Jesus Christ heals you." . . . Not only in the ministry of healing but in all the operations of the Spirit Jesus was believed to be continuing his work. The Spirit was indeed the Spirit of Jesus. The risen and regnant Lord had poured out the Spirit upon his disciples, and through the Spirit he exercised his sovereign

authority over them. In Acts every new development in the story is brought about by the guidance of the Spirit.[1]

This mission has continued through every age, right into the present.

THE HOLY SPIRIT AND THE HEALTHY BODY

The Holy Spirit sustains the life of faith as breathing sustains the life of the body, and these are related. In fact, the word *spirit* originally meant "breath," drawn from the Latin word for "breath," *spiritus.* The inspiration of the Holy Spirit and the respiration of the body are linked in that breathing connects us with the vital energy given by God, which is necessary for life.

It is widely known that in the biblical story of creation, human life begins when God breathes the breath of life into the dusty form of man. It is not so widely recognized that in the biblical view this animation is an ongoing activity. God sustains life through the spirit (see Job 34:14). And if God should take back his spirit, all flesh would perish and return to dust. Furthermore, as God continues to "breathe into" (literally, "inspire") the world, not only are humans sustained, but the "face of the ground is renewed" (Ps. 104:29-30).

This understanding of the spirit of God from the Hebrew tradition is assumed and expanded in the Christian view to include other elements, including healing, which is of special interest to us here.

Christian Tradition

Breathing, prayer, and meditation are linked in Christian practice. The Orthodox tradition (dating back to apostolic times but distinct from the Roman Catholic Church since the eleventh century) has connected breathing and the "Jesus

Prayer." The monks Callistus and Ignatius gave these instructions in the fourteenth century:

> The natural method of entering the heart by attention through breathing, together with saying the prayer: Lord Jesus Christ, Son of God, have mercy upon me. This method contributes greatly to the concentration of thoughts. . . . "You know, brother, how we breathe: we breathe the air in and out. On this is based the life of the body and on this depends its warmth. So, sitting down in your cell, collect your mind, lead it into the path of the breath along which the air enters in, constrain it to enter the heart together with the inhaled air, and keep it there. Keep it there, but do not leave it silent and idle; instead give it the following prayer: 'Lord Jesus Christ, Son of God, have mercy upon me.' Let this be its constant occupation, never to be abandoned. For this work, by keeping the mind free from dreaming, renders it unassailable to suggestions of the enemy and leads it to Divine desire and love."[2]

The story of an anonymous nineteenth-century wanderer who literally took this prayer to heart has become a classic under the titles *The Way of the Pilgrim* and *The Pilgrim Continues His Way*. Ironically, this practice, which has been carried on for centuries largely in monasteries, came to public attention in the twentieth-century best-seller by J. D. Salinger, *Franny and Zooey*. The novel traces the consequences of the use of this prayer through Zooey's study of other world religions in a way that leaves no doubt about its relevance to contemporary life. Ron Delbene, an Episcopalian priest, has developed this ancient breath prayer in a form that has force and practical usefulness in *The Hunger of the Heart*.

Thus Spirit may refer to the invisible force that both comes upon us from without, like the wind, and moves within us, like breath. The Spirit is both transcendent and immanent, a factor that is important to healing, wherein the Spirit of God works on the human spirit.

In the living organisms of the psychophysical self, breathing provides the oxygen that keeps the metabolic fire going, turning food into fuel. Because the body cannot store large quantities of oxygen, brain damage or death occurs if breathing is stopped for more than a few minutes. Breathing is part of the basic life process, as is the beating of the heart.

Other World Religions

Breathing is an activity of spirit as well as a physical necessity.

In the Hindu tradition, for example, Prana is at once the breath of life, the life force, and cosmic energy. Yoga is the widely known practice based on this understanding, which involves an elaborate system of breathing and other exercises.

In the Chinese tradition, which originated in Taoism, Chi is the name of the vital energy that brings health when flowing harmoniously through the body. When Chi is blocked, illness results. Various interventions may be called for to unblock this energy (exercises such as Tai Chi, acupuncture, or herbs), but exercising the breath is basic.

The Medical World

The interaction of breath and spirit also is found in the medical world. Breathing and the Holy Spirit participate in each other. This may sound more mystical than medical, but in fact it is both. To better understand this relationship and some of its implications for healing, let us briefly consider the work of renowned practitioners in the field.

Alexander Lowen is widely known as the creator of Bioenergetic Analysis and as a practicing psychoanalyst, researcher, and author. No psychoanalyst since Wilhelm Reich has worked more rigorously with the body than Lowen. It is striking, therefore, that he should title a recent major work *The Spirituality of the Body*, "an attempt to uncover health's spiritual face." In this work, Lowen focuses on grace as a criterion of health in order to understand emotional prob-

lems and to develop "the gracefulness that promotes health."
He writes:

> Spirit and matter are joined in the concept of grace. In theol-
> ogy, grace is defined as "the divine influence acting within
> the heart to regenerate, sanctify and keep it." It could also be
> defined as the divine spirit acting within the body. The divine
> spirit is experienced as the natural gracefulness of the body
> and in the graciousness of the person's attitude toward all of
> God's creatures. Grace is a state of holiness, of wholeness, of
> connection to life, and of unity with the divine. This state is
> also one of health, as we shall see.[3]

The importance of breathing is stressed throughout
Lowen's work. The first task of Lowen's own therapy was to
learn to breathe more deeply and to deal with the emotional
and physical blocks discovered in doing so.

In *Bioenergetics,* he sets forth the basis of his revolutionary
approach, which views the human personality in terms of the
energetic processes of the body. He writes, "Bioenergetics
aims to help a person open his heart to life and love. . . .
Breathing plays an important role in bioenergetics because
only through breathing deeply and fully can one summon
the energy for a more spirited and spiritual life."

In *The Spirituality of the Body* he devotes an entire chapter
to breathing and bioenergetic exercises to aid it. That chapter
concludes with these words:

> Natural breathing is a gift of God, who breathed life into our
> bodies. This is an opportune moment to return to the notion
> that breathing in, after all, is synonymous with inspiration.
> According to the dictionary, to inspire is to infuse someone
> with an animating, quickening, or exalting influence, which
> is just what the inhalation of oxygen does. We can sometimes
> breathe life into a person with mouth-to-mouth resuscitation,
> just as God is reputed to have done with the first man. I can
> also picture God, after creating the world, stopping to take a
> good breath, like any honest laborer. As he did so, I have no

doubt that he saw it was meaningful and right. As we breathe deeply, it is easy to feel how right the world is, how fair, how beautiful. We are inspired. How tragic it is, then, that so few people breathe freely and well.[4]

Leonard Laskow is a medical doctor who believes that "healing occurs naturally, and love heals." Laskow has developed these themes in a program he calls holoenergetic healing, which he spells out in his book *Healing with Love*. Like Lowen, Laskow stresses breathing in the healing process, building on the ancient traditions we have mentioned but adding Western scientific studies and laboratory research by himself and others. "Life is breathing" writes Laskow, and controlled breathing is a major factor in his work.

In his book, Laskow identifies nine key functions of breathing that make it a vital force in healing: nourishment, building energetic charge, directing attention, accessing information, altering and reflecting feelings and thoughts, shifting and reflecting consciousness, inducing resonance, and linking the conscious and unconscious minds.

In addition to discussing the physiology of breathing and presenting seven breathing exercises, he relates the medical significance of breathing to the spirit. He writes:

> The balancing breath links you with your spirit, and it helps to bring healing into the realm of conscious choice. . . . In those moments when we experience oneness and come into alignment with our source, or true nature, we no longer feel alone or abandoned. We are coming home, in resonance with our source. If we remain misaligned or separated from our source, we eventually become ill, which reminds us to come back into resonant unity. The essence of healing, then, is to become one with the source of our being.
>
> I like the way the Gospel of Thomas addresses the illusion of separation and duality and the unity of matter and spirit:

> Jesus saw children who were being suckled.
> He said to his disciples:

> These children who are being suckled
> are like those who enter the Kingdom.
> They said unto him:
> Shall we then, being children,
> enter the Kingdom?
> Jesus said to them:
> When you make the two one,
> and when you make the inner as the outer
> and the outer as the inner,
> and the above as the below,
> and when you make
> the male and the female into a single one,
> so that the male will not be male
> and the female not be female,
> then shall you enter the Kingdom. (Thomas 2.2-22)[5]

Breathing and healing are related in the work of the Stress Reduction Clinic at the University of Massachusetts Medical Center. This effective program shares with Christianity its profound concern for suffering while it draws on the Buddhist practice of mindfulness meditation.

Jon Kabat-Zinn, the founder of the Stress Reduction Clinic at the University of Massachusetts Medical Center and the author of *Full Catastrophe Living,* is "the end of the line" to whom medical colleagues refer their patients when there is nothing more they can do for them. At the heart of his treatment is the practice known as mindfulness meditation. Mindfulness is both a form of meditation and a way of life that seeks to keep one's consciousness alive to present reality. Seven attitudinal factors are the pillars of this practice: nonjudging, patience, a beginner's mind, trust, nonstriving, acceptance, and letting go.

According to Kabat-Zinn, mindfulness helps people deal with pain.

> [Mindfulness] allows you to learn from your own inner experience that pain is something you can work with, and that you can actually use pain to grow. Sometimes you have to learn

how to work around the edges of your pain and to live with it. The pain itself will teach you how to do that if you listen to it and work with it mindfully . . . meaning that when pain comes up in the body, instead of focusing on the breath, you just start breathing with the pain. See if you can ride the waves of the sensation. As you watch the sensations come and go, very often they will change, and you begin to realize that the pain has a life of its own. You learn how to work with the pain, to befriend it, to listen to it, and in some way to honor it. In the process of doing that, you wind up seeing that it's possible to feel differently about your pain. Sometimes, when you focus on this, the sensations actually go away.[6]

Mindfulness was pioneered in the West by Thich Nhat Hanh, a Buddhist monk originally from Vietnam who discovered its healing power in his own experience. He writes:

Years ago, I was extremely ill. After several years of taking medicine and undergoing medical treatment, my condition was unimproved. So I turned to the method of breathing and, thanks to that, was able to heal myself. Breath is a tool.

Breath itself is mindfulness. The use of breath as a tool may help one obtain immense benefits, but these cannot be considered as ends in themselves. These benefits are only the by-products of the realization of mindfulness.[7]

In the work of Alexander Lowen, Leonard Laskow, Jon Kabat-Zinn, and others, the respiration of the body is linked to the inspiration of the spirit for health and healing.

THE END OF THE ROAD

There comes a time when we can no longer breathe. What then? Death stands at the end of the road after all our efforts to be healed. We can go no farther in our present form. At some point our bodies can no longer function. No discussion of healing that denies this can be credible.

Pablo Picasso created a painting called "The End of the Road." The painting shows two long lines of people of every age and condition: young and old, rich and poor, erect and bent. They are all moving in the same direction. At the end of the road is the angel of death, white wings spread over his bleached skull.

All of us travel that road. There is no escape. At last each one of us, like those we love, come to the end of the road. Saddened though we are by this theme, we must admit that death is real. Although some writers are tempted to think otherwise, in the end the Bible does not deny death. The Bible acknowledges that all human beings come to the end of the road.

We know this is true of everyone else, but we have a terrible and difficult time admitting it about ourselves. Indeed, it is almost impossible for us to contemplate our own end. It is common for people to think that death is what happens to other people but not to them. Yet everyone carries the end of the world around in the form of his or her own death. This is what makes the subject at once so critically important and so difficult to face.

Every nation carries the end of the world around with it in the form of its own potential devastation. Every society carries the end of the world around with it in the form of its demise. Every civilization carries the end of the world around with it in the form of its decline and fall. We live for a moment in our lives, in our towns and cities, in our nations, in our world, in our galaxy as if we will live forever. We will not.

The Holy Spirit and Death

If the Christian faith did not recognize the reality of death, it would not be credible. If in the face of death someone would try to propose to us, "Ah, come on, don't worry about it. Everything is going to be all right. There really isn't any death; there's no pain; there's nothing to fear; everything is

104

beautiful," we would say, "Get away from me. I want nothing to do with you." That would be to deny the actuality that eats away at us and faces us with an undeniable pain. When the Christian faith affirms the resurrection of the body, we acknowledge that there could be no resurrection if there were no death. Although we are shocked by it, we recognize that this makes the faith more credible.

But if the Christian faith had only that to say, then we would not be comforted. The Christian faith recognizes the actuality of death but dares to affirm that there is more. There is death, but there is life beyond death. When we say, "I believe in the resurrection of the body, the life everlasting, and the communion of saints," we are affirming the belief that at the end of the road another road begins.

One day I was driving through the moors of England in a "mini"—a very small car in a very large landscape. I was lost in the magic of the landscape. Suddenly an enormous black rock loomed directly in from of me. I panicked. There seemed to be no way to avoid disaster. I hit the brakes, and hoped, and turned as sharply as I could to avoid crashing headlong into the rock. I skidded to the right on the road, which continued in that direction, although I could not see that before. I traveled on, shaken, but more than ever appreciative of my journey.

This incident has become a parable to me: I came to the end of the road. Another road I could not see before opened up to me.

When we think about the people who have been dear to us, who walk with us no more, we sense the sadness of coming to the end of the road. We miss them. Hardly a day goes by that I do not remember and mourn somebody. The longer we live, the more we are faced with the loss of our family and friends.

We feel the sadness at the end of the road; yet, we have that experience sometimes in our commonplace travels of coming down to the end of the road, thinking that we can't go any farther, and suddenly another road opens up.

If this is true in our most common experiences, surely it can be true in the most devastating experiences of our life. We come to the end of the road, but another road opens up before us and life goes on, different from before, but life goes on. If it goes on for us, then we can affirm in faith that it goes on somehow mysteriously for those whom we have loved but cannot see in the way we did before.

The grand experience on which this is based is what happened with our Lord. In that harsh and dreadful crucifixion, he certainly came to the end of the road; yet, days later he was alive! He was with the disciples. They knew his presence. They knew his love. They believed he was guiding them. He was present with them, in the breaking of bread, in the pouring of wine, and they remembered his words, "Do this in remembrance." In remembrance he was present, even as he is present today with us through the Holy Spirit.

The Resurrection of the Body

The resurrection of the body is both a future hope and a present reality. As a hope, the resurrection expresses a longing for a future in which the promise of the body is fulfilled beyond the limits of earth. As a present reality, the resurrection signifies the rising up from the deathliness of illness to fulfill that wellness that is possible within the limits of this life. When Jesus told the paralytic to rise up and walk, he was prefiguring resurrection "in the last days."

The Christian view of the resurrection of the body and life everlasting takes death with utter seriousness. One dies; one does not just "pass away." This flies in the face of sentimentality and the cosmetic side of the mortician's work which often seems to be to make the person in the casket appear as if nothing had happened. But death is real, and there is reason to weep.

Faith in the resurrection of the body and the life everlasting is faith that beyond this death there is more life. Faith knows that death is strong but that love is stronger. The resurrection and everlasting life are not simply continuities inherent in existence but acts of grace of which only God is capable. To live again is a gift of God no less mysterious or more merited than to live now.

Faith in the resurrection and the life everlasting appear most elusive to scientific scrutiny. Incredible as it may seem, life beyond death is one of the most scientifically studied and documented phenomena in the range of our study.

There is life. There is death. There is life beyond death.

For nearly two thousand years the church has witnessed to these three stages with secular society on the whole denying the third stage, especially in the modern scientific period. Now there is a trend to affirm the third stage with carefully documented studies that, to a remarkable degree, confirm the vision of the church.

Raymond A. Moody, Jr., pioneered in this field with his study of people who were declared clinically dead but returned to life. This study appeared in 1976 with the title *Life After Life.* Elisabeth Kübler-Ross saw his study in pre-publication form and revealed that she had been engaged in similar research, and her findings not only paralleled but duplicated Moody's. Kenneth Ring has conducted further research with rigorous scientific method and added significantly to the field in his books *Life at Death* and *Heading Toward Omega: In Search of the Meaning of the Near-Death Experience.*

Although there are wide variations in the types of persons and situations studied, there are remarkable similarities, including one major finding that is especially relevant here: At the core of near-death experiences "we find an absolute and undeniable spiritual radiance." In his book *Heading Toward Omega*, Kenneth Ring writes:

107

When we come to examine the core of full NDEs [near death experiences], we find an absolute and undeniable spiritual radiance. This spiritual core of the NDE is so awesome and overwhelming that the person who experiences it is at once and forever thrust into an entirely new mode of being.[8]

For the Christian, there is no denying the reality of life after death. Because of the resurrection, we can embrace death as a meaningful transition of life.

Embracing Death as Part of Life

Death is a reality. Yet death is more than the cessation of vital functions. To find the meaning of death, we see it as the end of life not only as its cessation but as its conclusion, the summing up of one's earthly existence. On the cross, Jesus cried out, "It is finished!" Surely he meant not only that his earthly life was over but that his work was complete. A poet wrote of this moment: "Love's redeeming work is done. . . . Fought the fight, the battle won."

Nothing that Jesus was or did could save him from death. But everything that Jesus was and did filled that death with meaning. Likewise, our task is not to escape death but to embrace it as part of life and fill it with meaning. We all have to die, but we do not have to die before we have truly lived and loved. Knowing the limits of life, we may attempt to deny them and assume a godlike superiority, but that never works. Alternately, knowing the limits of life, we may choose to live within them more passionately. Taking death seriously can help us enjoy life more fully.

The witness of Christian faith is not that there is no death but that there is life beyond death. The evidence on behalf of survival of human death presented in medical studies is overwhelming. Moreover, scientific data confirms the Christian vision of life after death to a remarkable degree.

HEALING INTO LIFE AND DEATH

In his book *Healing into Life and Death,* Stephen Levine says that an essential factor in all healing is love. He offers an example of this in the story of a woman called Hazel.

Hazel was hospitalized with cancer, which had infiltrated the bone and left her in "burning agony." Hazel was a very difficult person, a tough businesswoman, whose way of relating to others was so merciless that even her own children would not visit her because they had been pushed away so often. She had never met her grandchildren. Even her doctor and nurses were met with anger and scorn when they answered her bell.

After six months in the hospital, one night her pain was so great that it broke through all her walls of resistance. For one moment, perhaps the first in her life, she drew a single breath into her pain. She surrendered to her suffering and allowed it to move through her, without resisting. Later she said that in the moment when the troubled waters of her long resistance broke, she sensed that she was somehow not alone in her pain. She was joined by what she called "ten thousand people in pain." This experience broke her heart and brought her into contact with herself. She realized, "It wasn't my pain, it was *the* pain." She had shifted from the separate to the universal. Her heart had opened, and she had touched the suffering of the world with mercy and compassion.

Hazel's room then became the center of healing in the hospital for the next six weeks until she died. This was the place where love was so real and radiant that nurses would come there to spend their breaks. Soon her children came to visit her, responding to the warmth of her phone calls and her plea for forgiveness. Then her grandchildren, whom she had never met, sat next to her on her bed, playing "with Grandma's soft, sweet hands."

A picture of Jesus as the good Shepherd surrounded lovingly by children and animals was given to Hazel just a few days before she died. Hazel, whose life had been so hard and merciless, looked at the picture and with a cracking voice said, "Oh Jesus, have mercy on them, forgive them, they are only children."

According to Levine, Hazel's healing was one of the most remarkable ones he has ever seen. He writes: "For us it was an example of someone who seemed to have healed in a most profound manner, though she didn't stay in her body—a heart that opened incredibly, a deepening wisdom and a sense of participation in life which broadened with each day."[9] The very spirit of Jesus had entered that place of hurt and hatred and made of it a center of love and care.

This is the same Holy Spirit that is available to comfort us.

THE JOURNEY HOME

TOWARD HEALTH AND WHOLENESS

There is a wholeness to the Christian faith in relation to health. God the Creator endows us with wonderfully embodied minds and spirits. These marvelous creations enjoy pleasure but also experience pain and are threatened by illness and death. However, God in Jesus Christ joins us in our pain and pleasure to redeem and renew us. We are sustained by the Holy Spirit who brings the fullness of God to us and helps us to get back on the road. Eventually, we come to the end of the road as individuals and societies, but even here God is with us. As one road ends, another begins.

The power that heals is love: divine love expressed through creation, redemption, and sustenance interacting with human love in which persons care passionately and compassionately for God, neighbor, and self through awareness, acceptance, action, and affirmation. Confirmation is found in the experience of medical professionals such as Gerald Jampolski, who writes in his book *Healers on Healing:*

> For me, the common denominator in all healing is God. And because God and love are one and the same, the common denominator in healing is love. To heal and to be healed is to walk each day, each hour, each second with God. It is to recognize that God is our only true relationship. It is to

recognize every encounter with another person as a holy encounter, seeing only the holiness in that person.[1]

Love is the power that heals. This conviction has grown in me throughout this study. Again and again I have asked myself; what is the power that heals and how does it work? Again and again, the answer has been love working through loving. I have discovered that when I then ask what love is and how it works the answer comes that to love is to be aware, accepting, active, and affirmative.

This is obvious when I love another person. I become aware of that person in a heightened way. I am attracted by and to her or him. The person catches my eye and my heart. But that may be sheer attraction. Love means accepting other persons as we find them and not merely as they first appear. Love means showing my love by deeds of kindness, affection, and helpfulness. Love means affirming the other. Love means building them up in word and deed.

Love of God has these same dimensions. To love God is to pay attention to God in prayer and meditation, to look for God in the common things of life. It means to accept God as the ultimate reality in one's life and to trust God as the One into whose hand I finally fall. Love means action through service of God and of humanity. Without these acts of love, it is unreal. Love means affirmation of God. It means praising God in attitude and act, by the way one lives.

To love myself calls for awareness of myself. It means paying attention to my inner and outer being. It means being conscious of myself and not merely as roles I play or tasks I perform. Love means accepting myself as I am and not as I wish I were. It means accepting myself even though at times I do unacceptable things. Love means affirming myself. Love means believing myself to be of sacred worth whether I succeed or fail on any given day.

When I seek to love in this way, I discover how interrelated these loves are. I cannot accept myself when I am unacceptable, unless I know that God accepts me, even though I am unacceptable. And I cannot love God without finding God in the person who is in need. The love with which I love God is the love with which I love my neighbor and the love by which God loves me.

That divine love comes to me through creation, redemption, and sustenance every day of my life and calls me to love God, my neighbor, and myself. A triune God calls me to a triune love. Thus I discover that the process by which I live affirmatively and the process by which I am healed and the process by which I love are one. When I love the Lord my God with all my heart and soul and mind and strength, passionately, and my neighbor as myself, compassionately, then I am truly alive and well.

Journey is a metaphor often used for healing and for living. It captures the movement from illness to wellness with the sense of adventure along the way. But unlike ordinary journeys, our destination is not a specific place.

Paul pointed the way in 1 Corinthians 13:13: "Faith, hope, and love abide, these three; and the greatest of these is love." Many people are familiar with these words but few realize that the author actually draws his conclusion in the next verse, calling us to make love our aim. Everybody likes to hear about how great love is. But the real test comes when a person actually makes love the goal of life and seeks daily to move toward it.

Love is our destination. We do not often think about it this way. But in the light of the Bible and human experience, we may see that our ultimate destination is not a place at which we arrive but a love in which we participate.

Love is where we are going, and loving is the way. Love is our destination, and loving is the vehicle for getting us there. When we engage in an act of love, whether it is as large as a lifetime commitment or as small as taking out the garbage, love lives.

Love is true when it embraces God, self, and neighbor. "Lord, you have been our home in every generation," said the psalmist. And God is love.

Ironically, then, the goal of our journey to wholeness is already present in the first steps we take. In times of acute illness, we feel that the goal of health is far from us and will never be reached. But faith may discover the seed of redemption planted in the rocky soil of our suffering. We may not experience the removal of all symptoms or disabilities, but we may find the grace to go on in spite of them. Not to deny the suffering but to enter into it and seek its meaning may lead to renewal and recovery. When we begin to be aware, accepting, active, and affirmative rather than asleep, denying, passive, and negative, we are on the way home. And home is in every step of the journey we take.

When our journey of living becomes our journey of healing—which becomes our journey of loving God as Creator, Redeemer, and Sustainer—then these three are one for us, and we are home.

TOWARD A NEW ALLIANCE OF RELIGION AND MEDICINE

Like the journey of the individual toward health and wholeness, the journey of society toward a new understanding and practice of health and wholeness calls for a new alliance of religion and medicine.

The call of the medical community for spiritual resources for healing is one of the greatest opportunities for a new alliance since the Macedonians called out to Paul to come over and help. The health-care crisis in America and throughout the world may be met with a response that will positively affect every area of life when religion and medicine join forces.

Let us consider the implications of such an alliance for religion and the church, recognizing that the role of medicine must be more fully defined by its practitioners in relation to laypeople who are no longer simply patients but partners and affirming the positive contributions that have been and will be made by Western medicine with its many brilliant researchers and caring practitioners. Support for health-care professionals in their day-to-day work is called for. There is promise in ongoing research projects within Western medicine as well as in the special studies by the World Health Organization and the National Institutes of Health on alternative ways of healing. Much is to be expected from health-care professionals who master their specialty and are open to new directions.

If religion, and the church in particular, is to respond meaningfully to this call it must, no less than medicine, take major steps. These include the following:

Recover healing as central to Christian understanding. The concern for health and wholeness is at the center of the church's faith and mission. This is a major message of this book. However, this concern has been obscured and must be recovered if the church is to live by its own message.

Renew the historic ministries of healing. Healing has been not only a concept but a practice of the church since earliest times. The historic practices need to be reviewed and revitalized by contemporary understanding and commitment. This refers not only to specialized ministries but also to the healing dimension, implicit but often not explicit, in the ordinary life of the church. Worship, for example, is too often carried out by rote with the healing dimension of prayer ignored or trivialized. Holy Communion, in particular, must be renewed as the sacrament of suffering and redemption.

By historic ministries I mean those practiced since biblical times—such as worship, prayer, anointing with oil, and the laying on of hands—as well as those developed with the emergence of institutions and professions specializing in healing such as hospitals and chaplaincies, pastoral care, family counseling, and other contemporary forms of what has been long known as "the care of souls."

Relate healing and preaching anew. Jesus sent out his disciples to preach and to heal in one mission. Preaching and healing have now by and large become two completely different tasks in a way that diminishes both. The time has come to recover the organic relationship between them. Preachers as well as their hearers will benefit from this. There are signs of the failure of preaching to address many people today. Especially distressing is the rising rate of stress and burnout among pastors. Preaching has become so much an activity in and of itself that individuals who are excellent preachers may suffer from serious health problems, often psychological, that nullify their pulpit performance.

"Preacher, heal thyself!" is the first step in the rapprochement of preaching and healing. Revisioning homiletics for connections to therapeutic as well as rhetorical study is necessary. Training of pastors at the seminary and post-graduate level to be both preachers and healers will be a major step in this endeavor.

Research and develop emerging forms of health care. There is need for major research in the theory and practice of the new approaches to wellness to discern the church's role in the emerging situation. This would involve identification of goals, methods, issues, ideas, persons, and institutions engaged in the work and criteria for evaluating them. Development of plans based on this research would be a step toward discovering and/or creating alternatives. Medical research centers, theological schools, institutes, holistic learning sites, hospices, and local churches are among the obvious places to look.

The Third World is a not-so-obvious, but extremely important, setting for such study. In some of these places, radically new forms of community health care are coming into being literally from the ground up, involving basic environmental issues as well as sanitation, nutrition, and care for the ill. The

Jamkhed project in India is such a place. Plans are already underway to spread community-based health care programs in Bolivia and throughout Latin America. These projects have important messages for communities throughout the world where complex, very expensive high-tech medicine complicates itself beyond the reach of the people.

Participate in the hermeneutics of healing. The hermeneutics of healing will be a major task of this new alliance between religion and medicine. Hermeneutics is the art and science of interpretation, and it is potentially important in guiding how we interpret the signs and symbols of our illness and health. Traditionally, the data to be interpreted has been literary texts, but another kind of text may be one's spirit-body, and how that is interpreted is crucial to treatment and recovery.

For example, what is the primary datum to be treated? Is it a body part that may be infected or the person whose body part is infected? The answer will direct the treatment. If the person is the primary datum of treatment, then the person's worldview, philosophy, theology, and beliefs are relevant factors as well as the strictly medical factors.

Pain and suffering, often linked together, are not the same. What individuals experience as pain and how they try to get relief involves a vast network of sensations, perceptions, observations, assumptions, thoughts, and emotions. Interpretation is going on all the time, by patients and practitioners alike. Hermeneutics can help sort out the data, aid in treatment, and supply resources. To leap ahead, I suggest that the hermeneutics of healing is guided by these questions: How can illness build up the person's love of God, self, and neighbor? What is the message of this malady? What can we learn from this?

CHAPTER
EIGHT

PICTURES OF HEALTH

We sometimes say that a person is "the picture of health." Often such a person has an erect bearing and a glow about him or her, but this is not always the case. Let us look at some persons whose health has a direct relationship to the faith we are considering and who show afffirmative living in action.

ASHLEY

Ashley's story seems sad at first. He told me of an accident, deterioration of his body, acute pain, and little hope that he would get better. Then he told me about his wife. She had a rare disease in which the tissue in certain parts of her body died. She was bedridden most of the time, and there was no known cure for her.

I felt a terrible hopelessness, as if this sickness were something that would devour Ashley, his wife, and me, too, if I didn't get away from it. I could not believe that this was the same man I'd known as a bright and promising student. Then suddenly I became aware of my feeling and thought, "Wait! Is it his problem or yours that frightens you?"

Then I looked at Ashley and discovered an amazing thing. He did not seem upset by what had happened to him or what he was saying. In fact, his eyes were clear and untroubled, his voice expressive but calm. He seemed much more of a human being, more present, more substantial, more alive than he had seemed when he was much younger. I sensed I was in the presence of something deep and marvelous. What is it? I wondered.

I said something to express my sense of his strength, and he acknowledged that it had been very difficult. But then he said, "It's amazing what the Lord can do when you let him use you." Then he told me how his experience had driven him more deeply into life, had brought him and his wife closer together and closer to their children. Even in his work he had seen better things than he had been able to achieve before.

In our continuing conversation, Ashley has told me more of his journey of faith. It is a powerful story, still unfolding, and it represents the venture in faith. Here is how he described some of it to me:

When I wrote to you last, I was in bed for three weeks to little or no avail, so the next step was an epidural block on February 27 which was has given some relief. The neurologist explained that it will probably be the end of August before I am feeling 100 percent under the best of circumstances, which seems unlikely now because the program has been slow due to prolonged stress and my own drive to push ahead too quickly.

One lesson I have been trying to learn: "They who wait for the Lord shall renew their strength; they shall mount up with wings like the eagle, they shall run and not be weary, they shall walk and not faint" (Isaiah 40:31). A song on this theme ends with, "Teach me, Lord, teach me, Lord, to wait." I have sung that song many a day, over and over.

When [a former professor] lectured, it was certainly like listening to a sermon, and I often experienced—but most especially on one occasion—a surge of excitement, a sense of awakening, a dawning, a ray of light breaking through the darkness of my mind and soul. That one lecture was, in some ways, what I imagine John Wesley might have experienced at Aldersgate. The light that dawned for me was at once terrifyingly exciting, painful, and liberating. The light revealed both an excited rush of new hope and the painful truth of all the work that lay ahead, the wounds that needed healing, the levels of maturity to be reached—all in a blinding moment—a terrifying projection which has become, in retrospect, suffering and joy which have produced endurance and faith. There has been great suffering, but equal and even greater joy; and never, truly never, more of either than I could endure.

Since that experience in that classroom nearly twenty years ago, that knowledge that I am always becoming and never static, fixed, "done" has kept me going and has turned belief into a kinetic faith, a dynamic, life-giving assurance of things hoped for. That experience was a major breakthrough and a foundation stone in my faith, life, and ministry. Many, many other experiences too numerous to detail have followed which have been building blocks.

People who know what our trials have been in the past year ask, "How do you do it?" I can quite honestly say, "Because I have a Helper."

I wrote this poem during one of these experiences which formed a building block:

Discovery

Spring diminishes into Winter
Soft flakes drift down
And softly cover
The deep—bright vibrancy of life recovered.
Silently, impartially,
The hoary blanket swaddles
Half-lived moments,
Dreams unfulfilled.
Life-giving joy nods beneath the weight
    of the chill—warmth of winterdrear.

Fall-parched roots snatch frantically for
Some dim nourishing sip
Of yesterday's ecstacy.

Summer reveries hide behind
Icy tears.

Hope lies cradled in despair
No life left to give.

Somehow warm rays penetrate
The heart,
Thawing stranded surge.
Embers of expectancy rekindle
God's incarnate mystery.

"Hope lies cradled in despair" was another ray of light, an insight that arose out of a slowly growing faith, the Spirit of Truth penetrating the weight and darkness of pain of the mind, body, and spirit.

How distant those days are now. My life is so often flooded with light. The old wounds have been cauterized, and most are healed; some are still healing. The light is winning the battle with darkness. Oh, there are still very real moments of anxiety, even despair, anger, and frustration; but I am flooded with the knowledge and assurance of victory much more quickly and powerfully. I now know that I no longer carry burdens alone, nor am I seeking my own ends for my own glorification and self-satisfaction. I work hard. I love my work and find great satisfaction in it, but nothing of any consequence happens by my efforts alone. The only accomplishments of any consequence come only as I allow God to work through me, to use me as an instrument, a channel.

PENNY

Penny is a pilot who has never had an accident in an airplane but who knows what it means to crash and burn. Her story shows how faith in the Trinity is actually lived. Let her tell you about it:

My understanding of God has evolved over the years through an interplay between personal experience and biblical, theological, and historical sources. As I look over the years of my life, there are at least two, maybe three, times when everything seemed to change. Interestingly, these two or three shifts represent changes in theological perspective as well. I will call these three periods Creator, Redeemer, Sustainer. The Creator phase, my childhood and youth, could also be called the "playground" phase. As a suburban child of privilege, the side of God I saw was the creator. God was the maker of a marvelous creation. The world to be experienced. God was the bestower of all blessings— my family, the garden, the beach, the sky, the seagulls and the moon and the fireplace in the family home.

The Redeemer phase, from age nineteen to twenty-four, could also be called the "rebellion" phase. In one year, I was "converted" to Christianity, left home, became a flight instructor, and experienced a shift in key relationships. It was during this rebellion phase that the Redeemer side of the Trinity became prominent. Life all of a sudden had a good measure of pain, struggle, and confusion mixed in with the joy. I was a new Christian struggling to make my way in the world. During this time, Jesus became real to me as Savior and guide.

The Sustainer phase began at the age of twenty-four, when everything changed for me once again. In 1982, I entered seminary in New York and left the airport behind. The man I loved died suddenly of a heart attack on the weekend between orientation and classes. I was also afraid of New York City. My key relationships seemed to fade into significance, leaving me vulnerable to the "dark night of the soul." In this time of despair, my theological focus became that of the sustainer. In that time of pain and grief, God was comforter, and even when I could not be comforted, God was present; and that was enough "good news" to get me through. Gradually comfort gave way to healing, integration, and growth, bringing me full circle to "new life."

My life is full now, both socially and professionally. It's too soon to tell, but I may be embarking on a new phase, one I hope will be more trinitarian, more integrated.

JOHN UPDIKE

Some days are so dazzling it takes years to see them clearly. I keep remembering the conversation I had with John Updike at a wedding reception at the Regency. I couldn't believe that I was actually looking at John Updike, and that he looked so happy.

He looked like someone I had known in high school who was at the wedding of his best friend. Surely someone who had written what he had written should be visibly marked by suffering. Instead his face shone like an athlete after a winning game.

His appearance as a bright and winsome human being helped me overcome my awe of him as a writer, my sense that he had written out of the background and consciousness of my personal life more than any other writer, that he knew me, that we had covered much of the same ground inside and outside, and that he had rendered it into literature.

I told him how much I had appreciated his work, especially his statement on the Apostles' Creed. He seemed genuinely appreciative of that, as if people didn't say that to him all the time.

He told me how much he had appreciated the ceremony. He really meant it. I was embarrassed, but it gave me courage to say, "You know, John, I have sometimes thought that you have struggled with a call to the ministry."

"Oh, no, no," he said quickly, reddening slightly. "Oh, no." I thought he reacted too quickly and strongly, that I may have cut in too close, too fast. I went on to say how I had found his portraits of ministers critical but sympathetic, his reading of theology serious and astute, and his interpretation of life a theological one—that is, oriented to ultimate meaning with a passion for intimate events.

His face and bearing changed. He seemed more relaxed. "Yes," he said. "You're right, in a way."

There was a silence that said a lot. I had felt that he had a vocation and that it was a priestly and prophetic one, that he might even have considered the ministry as a young man but had taken that calling with him into writing and had become a priest of the imagination, going forth daily into the smithy of the soul to forge the immortal conscience of the race.

All this was going on in the silence. I didn't know what to say next. I didn't have to. Updike said, "How is your ministry going?"

I found myself telling him what I had never told anyone else; how I had come to New York with bright hopes and collided with dark reality; that the experience had been devastating to me and my family; that I was all right now but that the struggle was more difficult than I had expected it to be; that I still experienced moments of grace and sought to share them.

He responded compassionately. I'll never forget what he said, "I hope you don't get so bent out of shape that you don't recognize yourself."

His words were so prophetic and spoken with such compassion that they went right to the center I had almost lost. As we talked further, I could feel my forces begin to stir again.

In that moment John Updike ministered to me and gave me a fresh understanding of that ministry to which all Christians are called: to enter compassionately into suffering so as to communicate at the point of desperate need—the descent into hell—that there is One who cares.

This experience is valuable because of the healing wisdom John Updike shared with me. It also gives me a chance to acknowledge the contribution of artists and their arts to the healing process. I, who had fancied myself ministering to the artist, was once again ministered to by the artist. John Updike, Kurt Vonnegut, Jill Krementz, and a host of others help us to heal through naming our pain and illuminating our path by their lives and work.

This incident further shows that tremendously important acts of healing occur not only in operating rooms or doctors' offices but in quiet conversations in unexpected times and places. Healing would be aided if we were more open more often to the physician in the person with whom we are speaking.

A GROUP PHOTO

Pictures of health are not only of individuals. Healing often takes place in groups. Here is a group photo.

I was one of a group of ministers exploring our professional development in a small, but mixed, group, led by Pat Carlisle. Among us were males and females, young and old, black, white, and Hispanic: a fairly representative sampling of clergy for a small group. We soon selected the subgroups in which we would interact, and the seminar was underway.

Everything seemed to be going smoothly until the second day when the subgroups were discussed. One member confessed that she was unhappy with her group because her needs were not being met, and she wanted to change. She was a white female who had brought her toddler daughter to the seminar and into the group with two white males and one black male. She sometimes held her daughter, sometimes let her loose to play, sometimes handed her over to other members of the group, sometimes left her to sleep.

The group was surprised and hurt when this woman complained. We had been under the impression that we had tried to accommodate her, after she had introduced unusual strains into the process. We tried to adjust quickly to solve the problem by simply regrouping and going on with the announced agenda of the meeting. But the leader refused to treat the issue as merely logistical. Wisely he kept the group tuned in on the issues underlying the complaints and our responses.

We were willing to go deeper. As we did, layer after layer of issues was exposed: male-female, black-white, Hispanic-Anglo, older-younger, powerful-powerless, First World-Third World, urban-suburban, and so forth. As we confessed our thoughts and feelings, there were times when it appeared that the whole project would not work. But as we continued, defense after defense, wall after wall fell and a common ground emerged on which all could stand. What could have been merely another professional seminar became a deeply personal and healing experience.

When the breakthrough came, the leader exclaimed, "I feel like singing!" We sang a chorus:

> Father, I adore Thee,
> Lay my life before Thee . . .
>
> Jesus, I adore Thee,
> Lay my life before Thee . . .
>
> Spirit, I adore Thee,
> Lay my life before Thee . . .

That was the conclusion of the chorus as it had been taught. But the song did not end there. The woman who had brought her daughter continued, "Midwife, I adore Thee," and the group joined in, "Lay my life before Thee." Then a couple sang, "Liberator, I adore Thee," and we all sang, "Lay my life before Thee."

What had begun as a traditional chorus to God the Father, Son, and Holy Spirit had become an anthem gathering up new concerns without sacrificing the old. By this time we all were singing. Out of many voices came one song.

This event is a parable of where we are now and where we may be able to go. Many voices are crying out to be heard. There are conflicting claims and competing interests in our confessions of what most concerns us. Our traditions are being tested by a future that intrudes on us like a beautiful, noisy, laughing, crying, angry, sweet, sometimes soiled infant. If we try to deny this or ignore it or force one form of language upon our situation, we will not be able to discover the strengths within this situation.

But if we speak honestly from the deepest voice within us and listen with equal intensity to others, we will hear and create a richer song than we have ever sung before and give voice to a deeper faith than we have ever confessed before. The persons who began the song by singing of God as Father, Son, and Holy Spirit sang deeply and truly. Those who joined in the singing, adding the voices of feminism and liberation and opening the way for others, sang no less deeply and truly. Together the hymn of praise was deeper and truer than anyone or any group could have sung alone.

We do not live in a time when all the people agree on all the words for all our faith. We do live in a time when amid our different words an eternal music is still to be heard. It is my faith that if we sing genuinely and listen earnestly, we will give voice to a faith eternal as the One who inspires it and as timely as the persons who declare it.

It was no accident that the song that accompanied the healing and creativity of this group began with praise to the triune God. The Trinity for centuries has been the subject of such praise. Nor is it accidental that new verses were added, for this is the witness of our times.

The power of the Trinity lies not in its capacity to end debate and solve all conflicts, but rather to provide a center for differing claims about God and human experience, which leads us to the circumference of a full faith.

The power of the Trinity is the power of love. Whatever else the Trinity claims, it tells us of the God who loves by creating, redeeming, and supporting. If we view the Trinity as merely an exercise in logic or mathematics or even theology, we miss its meaning. The Trinity calls us to love God, self, and neighbor. A triune God calls us to a triune love.

HELP FOR THE JOURNEY

"Do you want to be healed?" is an intensely personal question, and how it is answered will vary with every individual. In the end, all must answer this question for themselves. However, it may be helpful to identify some specific tools or resources for integrating insights from this study into your life. These are varied in nature, assuming that imaginative exercises may reach those persons who are not so moved by argument and that some may be more experienced in practices such as meditation.

AFFIRMATIVE LIVING

Affirmative living, by which I mean a healthy way of life, is essential for anyone who wants to be healed. Anyone who wants to experience the power that heals should be helped by practicing the process of Awareness, Acceptance, Action, and Affirmation on a regular basis. While my view of these elements linked as a dynamic process is unique as far as I know, the elements are found in many traditions.

Begin by using this approach as a way to get an overview of your life and health, a "diagnostic tool" if you will. Carefully examine yourself to become aware of your wellness or illness; accept what you find; decide how you are going to treat yourself, whether with traditional or alternative means.

Find the source of your affirmation. Act. Take the steps necessary to move toward wellness.

Use this approach as a pattern for daily meditation practice (see chap. 1, "The Journey to Wholeness"). Focusing on affirmations will not in itself bring about change. But when they are genuinely "the faith factor" in an overall health regimen, they can be decisive.

Here are affirmations based on God's love as described in this book. Any of them may be used at any time as appropriate.

God's Love Creates

God is granting me life as a gift.
I am receiving my life as a gift.*
I am offering my life as a gift . . . to God . . . to others.*
Divine Love is working through me here and now.
I am one with my higher nature, and I have creative power.
I am taking care of the earth with God.
I am working together with God to create a new world.

* These may be practiced by breathing in on "Receiving my life as a gift" and breathing out on "Offering my life as a gift."

God's Love Redeems

Lord, I do love you now.
Lord, I trust my life to you.
Loving is living for me.
I can do all things through Christ.
Lord Jesus Christ, have mercy on me.
Light of my life, dawn on my darkness,
Christ, all things are mine, for I am yours.

God's Love Sustains

Come, Holy Spirit, come.
Lead me in thy way, O Lord.

All things rise in praise of you, Lord.
I am a child of the dawn.

No affirmation is limited to any one season, and some are especially durable, such as "Lord, thy will, not mine, be done," "Letting go of it all now," "I am walking humbly with you, Lord."

THE AFFIRMATION GROUP

A group may be formed to support you and others in living your affirmations. I lead a small group of eight to ten members who meet to share affirmations. If many more came, we would most likely form another group, since ten is large enough to offer variety but small enough to allow everyone to take part.

The purpose of the Affirmation Group is to affirm one another in our ongoing life of faith. It is a support group, not a therapy group, although aspects of it are like an encounter group. I lead the group by introducing a theme and assuring everyone a chance to take part. Any one of the members could lead the group in this way. Usually we begin with a prayer or meditation. The leader makes a brief statement on some aspect of affirmation. This is discussed, then the floor is open for anyone to share an affirmation and what she or he is discovering in seeking to live it. The members interact with one another in a supportive, nonjudgmental way. We close with a prayer circle and, of course, an affirmation.

A key to the group is having each member write out an affirmation (an index card works well), illustrate it with a simple symbol (shining sun, blooming flower, butterfly, etc.), and share it with the group. With everyone's permission, I photocopy the cards and make copies available to the group. Then we join in affirming one another in the group and in our personal devotions. For example, for the person who is af-firming more joy in life, symbolized by the sun, we may affirm: "God is granting (name) joy in life" and visualize that person shining in the light. Affirming one another in these ways has a powerful effect.

Based on my experience in this affirmation group, I recommend such groups as a means of support, healing, and growth.

EXERCISES FOR PERSONAL USE

Here are three exercises to help you gain access to God's love: Creating, Redeeming, and Sustaining, in that order.

God's Love Creates Me

This exercise is to help you discover the Creator's unconditional love for you in your body. Notice and write down the negative and positive thoughts you have about your body every day. Do this for several days and see if there is a preponderance of negative thoughts. If so, pick out the negative items and rewrite your list, placing a positive item after every negative item. Keep doing this every day until you notice the shift to a preponderance of the positive. Let complete, unalterable acceptance of yourself bring you peace.

God's Love Redeems Me

Close your eyes and picture your television set. You are tuned to CNN, and it's time for "Larry King Live." See the graphics with the huge mike, hear the thundering sound and the announcer saying, "Welcome to 'Larry King Live'! Tonight, Larry's special guest, Jesus Christ!" The camera focuses on Jesus. What does he look like? What expression is on his face? What is Larry's first question? What is Jesus' answer? What is the content and tone of his response?

Now it is time for listeners to call in. What questions do you have for Jesus Christ? Picture yourself placing the call and hearing Larry say the name of your hometown. What is your question? Imagine Jesus looking intently at you through the television set as you ask. What is his answer? How do you feel? Ponder the answer. What will you do with it?

Repeat this exercise from time to time. What questions would you like to ask Jesus Christ? Imagine him asking you questions he asked of others as recorded in the Bible. Imagine him asking you, "Do you want to be healed?" Imagine him saying to you, "Take up your life and live!"

God's Love Sustains Me: A Prayer

Visualize the symbols and movements as you pray:

O Master,

I come before you as did Nicodemus. I have much, but I have nothing. I am physically fed. I am spiritually malnourished. My life is too full of things and too empty of enduring purpose.

I feel warm. Hot. Feverish. Burning with conflict within and frustration without.

Now I feel a cool breeze across my face. I welcome its coolness, its freshness. The wind brushes my body from head to foot, bringing relief to all of me.

The wind of the Spirit moves within me now. It blows through the rooms of my memory, tossing hidden things onto the floor: my mistakes, my sins, my failures, my dirty laundry, my secret shame, my private guilt. They are all blowing about. It is painful to see them.

The wind grows stronger now. It catches up all this trash in a mighty whirlwind and carries it out the window—away, away, away, into the infinite sky. Away!

I am clean inside now. Cool. Calm. I am renewed. I have been born again in this spirit. I know that you love me, not just the world, but me so much that you gave yourself for me. Now, I love you and give myself for you and to others. To those close to me (visualize). *To those around me* (visualize).

The wind wraps itself around me now. Cooling me. Healing me. Setting me free at last. Thank you. Amen.

FORGIVENESS

Forgiveness is so important to healing that it is essential to find or create a way to express this need and turn in a new direction (confess and repent). Exercises alone cannot do this, but in the context of a healing process, they can be helpful. (See esp. the forgiveness discussions in Stephen Levine, *Healing into Life and Death* [New York: Anchor Books, 1987], pages 89-101; Leonard Laskow, *Healing with Love* [San Francisco: Harper, 1992], pp. 204-10; Gerald Jampolski, *Goodbye to Guilt* [Toronto: Bantam, 1985]; Joan Borysenko, *Guilt Is the Teacher, Love Is the Lesson* [New York: Warner Books, 1990]; and Christina Baldwin, *Life's Companion: Journal Writing as a Spiritual Quest* [New York: Bantam Books, 1991].)

HUMOR

Humor is a powerful healing agent, as we noted earlier. Take the medicine offered by "Doctor" Joey Adams in his books and columns. Norman Cousins found this helpful, as do I. "Doctor" Henny Youngman is highly recommended; his sense of humor keeps him going in his late eighties. See Youngman's autobiography, *Take My Life, Please* (New York: William Morrow, 1991). Find someone whose writings or performances make you laugh and give yourself a dose every day.

Look for humor in your own day-to-day experiences with people.

FAITH

Find and cultivate your own faith factor. This book stresses the health resources of Christian faith, but the world religions are rich in this regard. Expect this search to be rich, but not easy.

OTHER RESOURCES

Art is one of many other resources. There may be more healing in a poem or a painting or in music than in a medicine chest.

Books are such resources. I find the following especially helpful because they are penetrating, practical, and comprehensive and include lists of further resources: *The Spirituality of the Body*, Alexander Lowen; *Full Catastrophe Living*, Jon Kabat-Zinn; *Peace, Love and Healing*, Bernie Siegel; *The Mechanic and the Gardener*, Lawrence LeShan; *Fire in the Soul*, Joan Borysenko; *How Can I Help?* Ram Dass and Paul Gorman; *Compassion in Action*, Ram Dass and Mirabai Bush.

Common Boundary: The Interface Between Spirituality and Psychotherapy is the title of a magazine that brings together professionals and laypeople. The circulation office is at Common Boundary, 8528 Bradford Road, Silver Springs, MD 20815.

Centers of holistic health and education offer the chance for community as well as instruction. The Omega Institute in Rhinebeck, New York, and the Open Center in New York City are among those I find helpful. For catalogs and information write: Omega Institute, Lake Drive Rd., R.D. #2, Box 377, Rhinebeck, NY 12572; The Open Center, 83 Spring Street, New York, NY 10012.

James P. (Pat) Carlisle works with wellness for clergy and laity and may be reached at this address: The Center for Creative Church Leadership, Long View House, 1722 Niblick Avenue, Lancaster, PA 17602. Further information about resources, workshops, and retreats is available from the author at 21 James St., Babylon, NY 11702.

Make the commitment to take up your life and live. Here we come to a major paradox. On the one hand we are saying that we must assume responsibility for our health, but on the other hand we are saying that we are sick precisely because we have lost the power. This is our dilemma. How is it to be resolved? Theologically, by grace. God acts on our behalf to enable us to act on our own behalf.

Those who would argue for self-sufficiency are offended by this point of view. What power can be higher than that of the individual? Grace to them is superfluous.

Yet, the theological view finds an analogy in medicine itself. When an individual becomes ill and cannot heal themselves, the physician intervenes with a treatment that does not so much heal as enable persons to heal themselves.

In his book *The Springs of Creative Living*, Rollo May has pointed out that this is what happens in psychotherapy. Reliance on a higher power to overcome addiction is well known. Gerald G. May expands on this theme in *Addiction and Grace*.

Remember the paralytic who walked as recorded by John. Physically he may have been lame, but spiritually he was paralyzed (John 5). He had been aware of his problem for thirty-eight years, but he finally accepted his responsibility, acted by taking up his sleeping mat, and went on to affirm the grace that had made him whole.

The resources that were available to him are available to anyone who will take up his or her life and live.

NOTES

PREFACE

1. Bill Moyers, *Healing and the Mind* (New York: Doubleday, 1993), p. 142.

1. JOURNEY TO WHOLENESS

1. The story of Orel Hershiser's return was datelined Los Angeles, May 28, 1991, *Associated Press,* and appeared in the *New York Times* on Wednesday, May 29, 1991, under the headline "After 13-month Ordeal Hershiser Returns Tonight."

2. Richard Carson and Benjamin Shield, eds., *Healers on Healing* (Los Angeles: Jeremy P. Tarcher, Inc., 1989), p. 3.

3. Carl Jung, *Modern Man in Search of a Soul* (New York: Harcourt, Brace and World, Inc., 1933), p. 229.

4. D. H. Lawrence, *The Complete Poems,* eds. Vivian de Sola Pinto and F. Warren Roberts (New York: The Viking Press, 1971), p. 620.

2. AFFIRMATIVE LIVING

1. Joan Borysenko, *Guilt Is the Teacher, Love Is the Lesson* (New York: Warner Books, 1990), p. 1.

2. These elements are found in the work of Nathaniel Branden, among others. Although he does not stress affirmation or recognize self-transcendence, his work on self-esteem is nevertheless helpful. See his *The Psychology of Self-esteem* (New York: Bantam Books, 1969).

3. Judith Guest, *Ordinary People* (New York: The Viking Press, 1976), p. 1.

4. Bernie Siegel, *Love, Medicine, and Miracles* (New York: Harper & Row, 1986), p. 38. See also Siegel's *Peace, Love, and Healing* (New York: Harper & Row, 1989).

5. Joey Adams, *Live Longer Through Laughter* (New York: Stein and Day, 1984), foreword by Norman Cousins, pp. 7-8.

6. Alexander Lowen, *The Spirituality of the Body* (New York: Macmillan, 1990), p. 14.

7. Herbert Benson and William Proctor, *Beyond the Relaxation Response* (New York: Berkeley, 1985), p. 5.

8. Ibid., pp. 6-7.

9. Ibid., pp. 106-17.

10. See Ron Delbene with Mary Montgomery and Herb Montgomery, *Into the Light* (Nashville: The Upper Room, 1988). See especially chap. 2, "The Breath Prayer."

11. See Ira Progoff, *At a Journal Workshop: The Basic Text and Guide for Using the Intensive Journal* (New York: Dialogue House Library, 1975); *The Practice of Process Meditation: The Intensive Journal Way to Spiritual Experience* (New York: Dialogue House Library, 1980); and Christina Baldwin, *Journal Writing as a Spiritual Quest* (New York: Bantam Books, 1991).

3. TRINITY: THE POWER OF LOVE

1. John Donne, *The Complete Poetry and Selected Prose*, ed. Charles M. Coffin (New York: Modern Library, 1952), p. 252.

2. Lansing Lamont, *Day of Trinity* (New York: Antheneum, 1985), p. 70.

3. Ibid., p. 247.

4. See John Hersey, *Hiroshima* (New York: Alfred A. Knopf, 1985).

5. F. F. Bruce, *Interpreter's Dictionary of the Bible* (Nashville: Abingdon Press, 1962), p. 711.

6. Justo González views the Trinity as "the One who lives as three," which inspired me in his excellent *Mañana: Christian Theology from a Hispanic Perspective* (Nashville: Abingdon Press, 1990). Paul Tillich's work *Systematic Theology* looms large because it is profoundly trinitarian and concerned with healing. In *The Christian Understanding of God*, Nels F. S. Ferré developed a trinitarian approach based on love, which has a healing dimension. Karl Barth's *Dogmatics* is structured by the Trinity, although understood differently from Tillich or Ferré. Leonardo Boff spells out the trinitarian basis of Liberation theology in *Trinity and Society*. Matthew Fox presents a creative interpretation of the Trinity in *Creation Spirituality*. Sallie McFague shows how the Trinity illumines feminist and other issues in *Models of God*. Other works are worthy of serious consideration, including M. Douglas Meeks's *God the Economist*.

7. Augustine, *De Trinitate, The Basic Writings of Saint Augustine*, vol. 2, ed. W. J. Oates (New York: Random House, 1948), VIII.10.

8. David L. Miller, *Three Faces of God: Traces of the Trinity in Literature and Life* (Philadelphia: Fortress Press, 1986), pp. 43-44.

9. Thornton Wilder, *The Bridge of San Luis Rey* (New York: Washington Square Press, 1939), pp. 116-17.

4. GOD'S LOVE CREATES:
CARE FOR OUR HEALTH AND CARE FOR THE EARTH

1. Bernie S. Siegel, *Peace, Love, and Healing* (New York: Harper & Row, 1989), p. 4.
2. Ibid., pp. 30-33.
3. Donald W. Shriver, Jr., *The Lord's Prayer: A Way of Life* (Atlanta: John Knox Press, 1983), pp. 26-27.
4. Virginia Ramey Mollenkott, "Feminine Images of God in the Bible," *Circuit Rider* (June 1982), p. 13.
5. Sallie McFague, *Models of God: Theology for an Ecological, Nuclear Age* (Philadelphia: Fortress Press, 1987).
6. Norman Cousins, *Anatomy of an Illness* (New York: W. W. Norton and Co., 1979), p. 237.
7. Norman Cousins, *The Healing Heart* (New York: W. W. Norton and Co., 1983), p. 248.
8. Al Gore, *Earth in the Balance* (New York: Houghton Mifflin Company, 1992), pp. 367-68.

5. GOD'S LOVE REDEEMS:
JESUS CHRIST ON "LARRY KING LIVE"

1. Wilhelm Reich, *The Murder of Christ* (New York: Pocket Books, 1976), p. 26.
2. Nels F. S. Ferré, *The Christian Understanding of God* (New York: Harper and Bros., 1951), p. 184.
3. *A Kierkegaard Anthology*, Robert Bretall, ed. (Princeton, N.J.: Princeton University Press, 1946), p. 289.
4. Paul Tillich, *The New Being* (New York: Charles Scribner's Sons, 1955), pp. 7-9.

6. GOD'S LOVE SUSTAINS:
THE HOLY SPIRIT AND THE HEALTHY BODY

1. G. B. Caird, *The Apostolic Age* (London: Gerald Duckworth & Co., Ltd., 1972), pp. 64-66.
2. *Writing from the Philokalia on Prayer of the Heart*, trans. from the Russian by E. Kadloubovsky and G. E. H. Palmer (London: Faber and Faber, Ltd., undated), p. 192.
3. Alexander Lowen, *The Spirituality of the Body* (New York: Macmillan, 1990), pp. xiv, 52-53.

4. Alexander Lowen, *Bioenergetics* (New York: Penguin Books, 1977), pp. 43-44.

5. Leonard Laskow, *Healing with Love* (San Francisco: Harper, 1992), p. 107.

6. Bill Moyers, *Healing and the Mind* (New York: Doubleday, 1993), pp. 119-20.

7. Thich Nhat Hahn, *The Miracle of Mindfulness* (Boston: Beacon Press, 1975, 1976), p. 23.

8. Kenneth Ring, *Heading Toward Omega: In Search of the Meaning of Near-Death Experiences* (New York: William Morrow and Company, 1984), p. 50.

9. Stephen Levine has written two accounts of this woman identified as Hazel. The fuller version appears in *Healing into Life and Death* (New York: Anchor Books, 1987), pp. 11-14. The other appears in *Healers on Healing*, eds. Richard Carlson and Benjamin Shield (Los Angeles: Jeremy P. Tarcher, 1989), pp. 196-99.

7. THE JOURNEY HOME

1. Gerald Jampolski, *Healers on Healing*, eds. Richard Carlson and Benjamin Shield (Los Angeles: Jeremy P. Tarcher, 1989), p. 154.